Sleep Rituals
The Pleasure of Sleeping Well

Avelyn Skor

AHZURIA

Original Title: *Sleep Rituals – The Pleasure of Sleeping Well*

This is a non-fiction work that explores practices and concepts in the field of well-being and sleep health. Through a grounded and sensitive approach, the author offers practical and transformative pathways to restore rest and reshape our relationship with sleep.

1st Edition

Production Team

Author: Avelyn Skor
Editor: L. A. Santos
Cover: Studios Booklas / Mira Devane
Consultant: Hektor Alvien
Researchers: Elira Moss / Taren Hov / Juno Kells
Typesetting: Narek Vinz
Translation: Cyra Lommen

Publication and Identification

Sleep Rituals – The Pleasure of Sleeping Well
Ahzuria.com, 2025
Categories: Health & Well-being / Sleep Neuroscience
DDC: 613.79 — Sleep and Rest
CDU: 613.743 — Sleep hygiene. Restorative practices.

Prologue

You're not sleeping as you should. And you know it.

It doesn't take much to realize: that weariness coffee can't fix. The fragile mood, the foggy thoughts, the feeling of always being one step behind your own life. Maybe you've learned to normalize this discomfort—after all, who sleeps well these days?

But what if I told you this silent unease isn't normal? That there's something behind this persistent fatigue, something deeper than it seems? And that this book is the map that can lead you back to a forgotten territory: true rest.

"Sleep Rituals" is not just another book about insomnia. It's a silent manifesto against the culture of exhaustion. A work that doesn't shout, but awakens. That doesn't offer ready-made formulas, but invites the reconstruction of something essential: your relationship with repose.

Avelyn Skor, with rare sensitivity and depth, charts a path in this book that goes from the science of sleep to the human soul. Each chapter is a layer peeling away the belief that sleeping well is a privilege for the few—revealing, with almost surgical precision, that restorative sleep is within reach for anyone willing to change how they live... and breathe.

It's not about turning off the lights and hoping the body cooperates. It's about deconstructing what they've done to your nights. Artificial light, digital addictions, the glorification of constant performance: all this has been carefully analyzed in this work and elegantly exposed. Here, there's no cold technicality or empty self-help. There's method. There's ritual. There's truth.

As you turn the pages, you'll realize that sleep isn't just a biological stage—it's a state of reverence. A return to your center. A ritual of reconnection with what is most authentic in you: stillness. This book teaches how to build an intimate sanctuary, where the body not only rests but is reborn. It teaches that sleeping isn't shutting down, it's surrendering. It isn't stopping, it's aligning.

Through ancestral practices, neuroscientific evidence, and accessible guidance, Avelyn gives back to the reader something modernity has stolen: the *license to rest* without guilt.

And make no mistake: this isn't just a book for insomniacs. It's for those who feel life has lost its rhythm. For those who wake up more tired than they went to sleep. For those who suspect, deep down, that there's a lighter—and more lucid—way to live. And that this way begins with the simple, yet powerful, act of closing your eyes in peace.

You'll discover that every gesture before sleep—turning off a light, silencing a noise, inhaling an aroma—can become a key. That there are cycles within your body crying out for balance. That sleep is a portal, and crossing it consciously can transform more than just your nights: it can rescue your emotional sanity, your mental clarity, your physical vitality.

In a world that teaches us to win through effort, *Sleep Rituals* teaches us to win through rest.

Reading this book isn't just consuming content. It's an act of courage. Courage to break free from the fatigue that has become an identity. Courage to restore what has been neglected. Courage to say: *I deserve to sleep well.*

So, if there's something inside you yearning for more lightness, more silence, more wholeness... you've found the right place. But be warned: this book doesn't serve haste. It demands surrender. And it rewards with depth.

Breathe deeply. Slow down. Read with your body, not just your eyes. And prepare to return to a place you may have drifted far from: yourself, at peace.

Summary

Systematic Index

Chapter 6: Concept of Sanctuary - Introduces the idea of transforming the bedroom into a dedicated sanctuary for repose by intentionally managing lighting, organization, air quality, temperature, textures, aromas, and sound.

Chapter 7: Sleep Hygiene - Details a set of daily practices and behaviors, such as maintaining schedule regularity, managing light exposure, creating wind-down routines, and adopting mindful dietary habits, to naturally promote better sleep quality.

Chapter 8: Limiting Beliefs - Addresses ingrained cultural and personal beliefs that hinder rest, such as equating sleep with laziness or unproductivity, and offers strategies to identify and reframe these notions.

Chapter 9: Sleep in History - Contrasts modern views of sleep with the more integrated, respectful, and sometimes sacred perspectives held by ancient and traditional cultures, highlighting sleep's perceived role in healing and spiritual connection.

Chapter 10: Introduction to Sleep Tourism - Presents the emerging trend of sleep tourism, where specific destinations and programs are designed to optimize rest, offering inspiration for intensive sleep care.

Chapter 11: The Nightly Ritualization - Emphasizes creating a consistent sequence of calming pre-sleep actions (like warm baths, aromatherapy, light reading, gentle music) to condition the brain and nervous system for relaxation and sleep.

Chapter 12: Conscious Breathing - Explores techniques like the 4-7-8 breath, alternate nostril breathing, and diaphragmatic breathing as tools to regulate the nervous system, reduce anxiety, and facilitate the transition to sleep.

Chapter 13: Muscle Relaxation - Describes progressive muscle relaxation, a technique involving tensing and releasing specific muscle groups, to dissolve physical tension and promote deep bodily tranquility conducive to sleep.

Chapter 14: Sounds and Silences - Discusses managing the auditory environment through silence (using earplugs or soundproofing) or calming sounds (like white noise, nature sounds, or soft music) to mask disturbances and induce relaxation.

Chapter 15: Inducing Aromas - Introduces aromatherapy using essential oils like lavender, chamomile, or sandalwood, explaining how scents can influence the limbic system to calm the nervous system and promote sleep.

Chapter 16: The Power of Light - Details the impact of light on the circadian rhythm and melatonin production, advocating for maximizing natural light during the day and minimizing artificial (especially blue) light at night.

Chapter 17: Temperature and Texture - Explains the importance of maintaining a cool room temperature (around 18-21°C) and choosing breathable, comfortable sleepwear and bedding (natural fibers) for optimal thermoregulation and sensory comfort.

Chapter 18: Nutrition and Sleep - Addresses the bidirectional relationship between diet and sleep, highlighting tryptophan-rich foods, magnesium sources, and calming teas, while warning against caffeine, alcohol, heavy meals, and sugar near bedtime.

Chapter 19: Visualization Techniques - Introduces using guided imagery of peaceful scenes or journeys to calm mental agitation, interrupt anxious thoughts, and activate the relaxation response by engaging the mind creatively.

Chapter 20: Nightly Writing - Proposes writing (free-form journaling, gratitude lists, or to-do planning) before bed as a method to externalize worries, process emotions, and clear the mind for greater tranquility.

Chapter 21: Nightly Meditation - Presents meditation practices (mindfulness of breath, body scan, observing thoughts) suitable for bedtime to train attention, reduce reactivity to thoughts, and cultivate inner calm.

Chapter 22: Falling Asleep with Awareness - Integrates previously learned tools into a conscious practice of transitioning to sleep, emphasizing recognizing drowsiness cues and orchestrating nightly rituals with mindful intention.

Chapter 23: Sleep as Therapy - Views quality sleep as an active therapeutic process for emotional restoration, mental clarity, nervous system strengthening, and support in overcoming conditions like depression and anxiety.

Chapter 24: Cycles and Seasons - Discusses how sleep needs and patterns naturally fluctuate with external cycles (seasons, daylight changes) and internal rhythms (hormonal cycles, life stages, stress levels), advocating for flexibility and adaptation.

Chapter 25: The Inner Journey - Explores the symbolic dimension of sleep as a nightly voyage into the unconscious, where dreams and subtle sensations can offer insights for self-knowledge and integration.

Chapter 26: Sleep Diary - Recommends keeping a dedicated diary to track sleep patterns, related habits, and subjective quality, serving as a tool for self-awareness, pattern identification, and monitoring progress.

Chapter 27: Sleep and Creativity - Highlights the connection between sleep (especially REM) and creativity, explaining how rest consolidates ideas, fosters unexpected connections, and aids problem-solving.

Chapter 28: Mini-Sleep Retreats - Suggests creating intentional periods of intensive rest at home (e.g., weekends) by minimizing stimuli and maximizing relaxation practices to reset the system and recover energy.

Chapter 29: Sleep Tourism - Revisits sleep tourism as an expanding field offering specialized destinations and therapies, inviting reflection on integrating rest-focused care into all travel experiences.

Chapter 30: The House of Sleep - Extends the sanctuary concept to the entire home, proposing cultivating an atmosphere of calm, organization, and respect for rest in common areas and family routines.

Chapter 31: Autonomy and Choices - Synthesizes the book's learnings, empowering the reader to become their own guide by integrating self-knowledge, body listening, and coherent habits to make conscious choices about sleep.

Chapter 32: Sleep Ceremony - Proposes creating a personal symbolic ceremony to honor the learning journey, celebrate progress, and affirm the ongoing commitment to cultivating the art of sleeping well.

Chapter 1
The Value of Sleep

Nightly rest, that silent interlude punctuating our active lives, holds a value often underestimated in the hustle and bustle of everyday life. We tend to view sleep as a necessary pause, perhaps even a dispensable luxury sacrificed for productivity or extended leisure. However, this perspective overlooks a fundamental truth: sleeping is one of the most essential biological functions for our existence, a pillar as vital as breathing, eating, or drinking water.

It's not merely about switching off consciousness for a few hours; it's an active, complex, and deeply restorative process that reverberates through every cell in our body and every thought we form. Recognizing and honoring the value of sleep is the first step toward a fuller, healthier life, connected to our own nature.

The benefits of deep, restorative sleep extend across all dimensions of our being. Physically, it's during sleep that the body performs crucial maintenance and repair tasks. Muscles recover from daily exertion, tissues regenerate, and the immune system strengthens, producing cytokines essential for fighting infections and inflammation. A well-slept night acts as a true balm for the body, preparing it for the next day's challenges with renewed vigor. Our skin reflects this renewal, as does our general disposition for movement and physical activity. Ignoring this intrinsic need is like trying to run a marathon without proper training; the body eventually protests, signaling its exhaustion.

Mentally, sleep plays an irreplaceable role. While we sleep, the brain doesn't rest passively; it works diligently to consolidate memories, process information acquired during the day, and clear accumulated metabolic waste, such as the beta-amyloid protein associated with the development of neurodegenerative diseases. It's as if the mind undergoes a nightly cleanup, organizing files, discarding the irrelevant, and strengthening important neural connections. This nocturnal activity translates into a greater capacity for concentration, learning, and problem-solving during wakefulness. A rested mind is a clearer, more agile, and creative mind, capable of tackling intellectual challenges more effectively and with less effort.

On an emotional level, the impact of sleep is equally profound. Adequate rest regulates neurotransmitters linked to mood, such as serotonin and dopamine, helping to maintain stable emotional balance. REM sleep, in particular, seems crucial for processing emotional experiences, allowing us to better cope with stress and anxiety. When we sleep well, our emotional resilience increases; we become more patient, empathetic, and capable of managing our reactions to adversity. The sense of well-being that accompanies a good night's sleep is no mere coincidence; it's the direct result of biochemical and neurological processes that restore our ability to feel and interact with the world more positively and balancedly.

Conversely, sleep deprivation, even if partial or sporadic, triggers a cascade of negative consequences. The body, deprived of its essential recovery time, enters a state of alert, raising levels of cortisol, the stress hormone. This chronic stress not only generates tension and irritability but also weakens the immune system, making us more susceptible to infections and diseases. Lack of sleep is associated with an increased risk of cardiovascular problems, type 2 diabetes, obesity, and other chronic conditions that compromise quality of life and life expectancy. The body simply cannot operate at its optimal level without adequate rest; forcing it to do so incurs a debt that, sooner or later, manifests in our health.

Productivity, so valued in modern society, is paradoxically one of the first victims of sleep neglect. A tired mind struggles to concentrate, memory fails, decision-making becomes slower and prone to errors, and creativity diminishes. Trying to compensate for lost sleep with more hours of work or study is an ineffective and counterproductive strategy. Performance plummets, and the quality of work done under exhaustion rarely compensates for the effort expended. Recognizing that rest is an integral part of sustainable productivity is fundamental to breaking cycles of burnout and frustration. A rested professional is not only more efficient but also more innovative and collaborative.

Mood is another sensitive indicator of our sleep quality. Poorly slept nights often result in days marked by irritability, impatience, and a more pessimistic outlook on life. Minor setbacks can seem insurmountable, and the ability to handle the emotional demands of daily life is compromised. This mood alteration affects not only the individual but also their interpersonal relationships at work, in the family, and in social life. The emotional instability generated by lack of sleep can create a vicious cycle, where anxiety and stress make falling asleep even more difficult, perpetuating the problem.

Memory, that essential faculty for learning and identity itself, intrinsically depends on sleep. During the different sleep stages, especially slow-wave sleep and REM sleep, the brain actively works on memory consolidation, transferring information from the hippocampus to the prefrontal cortex for long-term storage. Sleep deprivation interferes with this vital process, making it harder to retain new information and access existing memories. Studying or working late, sacrificing sleep hours, can actually impair the learning and performance one seeks to achieve.

Finally, longevity and quality of life over the years are closely linked to our sleep habits. Consistent research shows that sleeping well and sufficiently contributes to healthier aging, reducing the risk of cognitive decline and age-related diseases. Caring for sleep is, therefore, a long-term investment in one's own health and well-being, a self-care practice that yields dividends throughout life. It's not a hedonistic pursuit of comfort, but a fundamental biological need that sustains our vitality and our capacity to live fully.

Cultivating a respectful relationship with sleep is, above all, an act of self-understanding. As we deepen our knowledge about the multifaceted impacts of nightly rest, we realize that neglecting it is neglecting ourselves on deep levels—physical, mental, and emotional. The culture of haste and constant performance has taught us to see rest as an interval between achievements, when in fact it is an intrinsic part of the achieving process itself. Sleeping well is not a sign of weakness or indulgence, but of wisdom—the wisdom of understanding that consistency and balance overcome exhaustion and continuous sacrifice.

Re-educating our routine to value sleep requires a paradigm shift, especially in a world that romanticizes relentless productivity. This involves establishing nighttime rituals, respecting schedules, disconnecting from artificial stimuli, and creating an environment conducive to rest. Small gestures, like dimming the lights, silencing the phone, or reading quietly before bed, signal to the body that it's time to slow down. Over time, these habits shape a new relationship with sleep—not as an end of the journey, but as a sacred space of regeneration that prepares us to be reborn each dawn with more clarity, energy, and presence.

By recognizing the vital importance of sleep, we commit to taking better care of ourselves. It is in this commitment that a more conscious and sustainable existence is built. Ultimately, sleeping well is a way of loving life—in its entirety—and ensuring that we are fully capable of living it with lucidity, health, and fullness.

Chapter 2
Understanding the Cycle

Entering the universe of sleep is like exploring a vast and mysterious territory that reveals itself in distinct cycles and phases, each with its specific function in maintaining our overall balance. Often, the frustration of waking up tired, even after hours in bed, lies precisely in the lack of knowledge about this nocturnal architecture. It's not enough just to close our eyes and wait for dawn; the brain and body need to transition harmoniously through a sequence of stages that, together, make up what we call the sleep cycle.

Understanding this dynamic is not merely an intellectual exercise but a fundamental key to unlocking the secrets of truly restorative rest, where quantity and quality meet to nourish body, mind, and spirit.

A night's sleep is not a monolithic block of unconsciousness. On the contrary, it is woven from cycles that repeat, on average, every 90 to 110 minutes. Within each cycle, we pass through different stages, classified as NREM (Non-Rapid Eye Movement) sleep and REM (Rapid Eye Movement) sleep. NREM sleep, in turn, is subdivided into three phases: N1, N2, and N3, representing a progressive deepening of rest. Each of these stages plays vital and complementary roles, ensuring that the body's diverse recovery needs are met. The beauty of this process lies in its complexity and its almost choreographed precision, a neurological ballet that occurs while we are, apparently, inactive.

The first stage, N1, marks the transition between wakefulness and sleep. It's that fleeting moment when we feel our eyes grow heavy, muscles relax, and consciousness begin to drift. In this light stage, we can still be easily awakened by noise or external stimuli. Brain activity slightly decreases, and we might experience sensations of falling or sudden muscle jerks, known as "hypnic jerks." Although short, this phase is the gateway to deeper rest. It's the initial invitation for the body and mind to start slowing down, gradually abandoning the alert state of wakefulness. People who nap quickly during the day usually only enter this superficial stage.

Soon after, we dive into stage N2, which occupies most of our total sleep time, about 45% to 55%. Here, sleep becomes more stable. Heart rate and body temperature decrease, and brain activity shows characteristic patterns called "sleep spindles" and "K-complexes," indicating a more significant disconnection from the external environment. Although it's still possible to be woken up, awakening is not as easy as in N1. Stage N2 is crucial for consolidating motor skills and for the general maintenance of rest, serving as an important base before and after the deeper phases and REM sleep. It's a period of fundamental rest, where the body truly begins to disengage from the day's activities.

The next phase, N3, is known as slow-wave sleep or deep sleep. This is the most restorative stage for the physical body. Brain activity drastically decreases, dominated by delta waves, which have low frequency and high amplitude. Breathing and heart rate reach their lowest levels, and muscles become completely relaxed. It's during N3 that most muscle recovery, tissue growth and repair, immune system strengthening, and the release of important hormones, like growth hormone, occur. Waking someone during this phase is difficult, and if it happens, the person usually feels disoriented and groggy for some time. The quality and quantity of N3 sleep are essential for feeling physically refreshed in the morning. Without it, the feeling of physical fatigue persists.

After progressing through phases N1, N2, and N3, the cycle usually returns briefly to N2 before entering the most intriguing stage: REM sleep. This stage is characterized by intense brain activity, similar to wakefulness, with rapid eye movements under closed eyelids – hence the name. Breathing and heart rate become irregular, and the body's muscles, except for the eyes and diaphragm, become temporarily paralyzed, a safety mechanism that prevents us from physically "acting out" our dreams. It's in REM sleep that the most vivid and narrative dreams occur. This phase is fundamental for memory consolidation, especially procedural memory (the "how-to" of things) and emotional memory. Processing emotional experiences, regulating mood, and developing creativity are strongly associated with adequate REM sleep.

Throughout the night, these NREM-REM cycles repeat several times. Early in the night, periods of N3 sleep (deep sleep) tend to be longer, prioritizing physical recovery. As the night progresses, REM sleep stages become progressively longer and more frequent, especially in the final hours before waking, focusing more on mental and emotional recovery. This cyclical architecture ensures that both physical, cognitive, and emotional needs are met in a balanced way.

Frequent sleep interruptions, whether due to nighttime awakenings or very short sleep, fragment this structure and prevent us from properly completing all necessary stages. This is where the answer lies for the feeling of morning fatigue, even after sleeping for a reasonable number of hours. If sleep quality is poor – with many awakenings, difficulty reaching deep sleep (N3), or insufficient REM sleep – the rest will not be truly restorative. We can spend eight hours in bed, but if most of that time is spent in light stages (N1 and N2) or if the cycles are constantly interrupted, we will wake up as if we had slept much less. Factors such as stress, anxiety, chronic pain, use of certain substances, or even an inadequate sleep environment can compromise the natural progression through these essential stages.

Understanding the natural mechanisms of sleep and the function of each stage empowers us to look beyond the clock. The question is not just "how much" we sleep, but "how" we sleep. This awareness is the foundation for the changes we will explore later. By identifying the potential thieves of our sleep quality, we can begin to implement targeted strategies to protect and optimize each phase of this vital cycle. Knowing that the body needs time to repair muscles in deep sleep and that the mind requires REM sleep to process emotions and consolidate learning transforms our perception of the act of sleeping.

Delving into the structure of sleep sheds light on invisible, yet crucial, aspects of our health. When we understand that each nocturnal phase fulfills an irreplaceable role, we begin to value not only the duration of sleep but also its fluidity and continuity. It is in this symphony of rhythms and transitions that the body finds fertile ground to heal, the mind to reorganize, and the emotional self to stabilize. The wisdom of the sleep cycle lies not only in its existence but in how it reflects the body's intelligence in keeping us whole, even during apparent inactivity. Ensuring this cycle occurs without interruption is, therefore, an act of cooperation with our own biology.

This understanding also casts new light on what we call "insomnia" or "light sleep." The problem isn't always the quantity of hours slept, but rather the fragmentation of stages or the difficulty in reaching the deeper ones. Often, seemingly harmless daily habits – like excessive screen use before bed, heavy dinners, or irregular routines – silently sabotage the complexity of this cycle. When we look at sleep from this perspective, we realize that improving it requires not just more time in bed, but a re-education of our patterns and stimuli. Healthy sleep is not just an outcome, but a construction that begins long before turning off the lights.

It's at this point that understanding turns into action. By learning to recognize and respect the sleep cycle, we take the first step towards restoring confidence in rest as a transformative experience. Sleeping well ceases to be a matter of luck and becomes a natural consequence of conscious choices. And with this new perspective, each night holds the potential to be a silent and regenerating journey—a process of reconnecting with what silently sustains everything we are during the day.

Chapter 3
Sleep and Health

Understanding sleep as an active, cyclical process essential for daily restoration paves the way for an even deeper realization: nightly rest is one of the master pillars upon which our integral health is built. It's not an isolated component, but a central axis that interconnects with and directly influences the systems governing our physical, mental, and emotional well-being. Investigating the intrinsic relationship between sleep and health is like discovering the invisible threads that weave the tapestry of our vitality. Therefore, taking care of sleep transcends the quest for a more energetic awakening; it becomes a fundamental act of maintaining and strengthening the very temple we inhabit: our body.

The immune system, our first line of defense against invading agents, heavily depends on the quality of our sleep. During nightly rest, especially in slow-wave sleep (N3), the body intensifies the production and release of cytokines, essential proteins that help promote sleep and combat inflammation, infections, and trauma. Sleep deprivation, even moderate, compromises this production, weakening the immune response and making the body more vulnerable to diseases, from common colds to more serious conditions. Studies consistently show that people who sleep less have a diminished immune response to vaccines and greater susceptibility to infections. Sleeping well acts as a true tonic for our natural defenses, strengthening our ability to resist and recover from external and internal aggressions.

Hormonal balance, which governs countless vital functions from growth to mood and appetite, is also profoundly influenced by the sleep-wake cycle. Crucial hormones are released in rhythmic patterns over 24 hours, and many of these release peaks occur during sleep. Growth hormone, vital for cellular and muscle repair, is predominantly secreted during deep sleep. Leptin and ghrelin, hormones that regulate appetite and satiety, also have their levels adjusted during sleep. Sleep deprivation disrupts this delicate hormonal orchestra, potentially leading to an increase in ghrelin (which stimulates hunger) and a decrease in leptin (which signals satiety). This imbalance contributes to increased appetite, especially for high-calorie foods, and is associated with a higher risk of weight gain and obesity. Cortisol, the stress hormone, also has its rhythm altered by lack of sleep, remaining elevated for longer periods and contributing to a state of chronic tension.

Cardiovascular health, a cornerstone of longevity, finds an indispensable ally in sleep. During normal sleep, blood pressure and heart rate decrease, allowing the cardiovascular system to rest and recover from the day's stress. Chronic sleep deprivation, however, keeps these parameters elevated for longer, overloading the heart and blood vessels. This condition is associated with an increased risk of hypertension, heart disease, heart attacks, and strokes. Insufficient sleep also contributes to systemic inflammatory processes and insulin resistance, additional cardiovascular risk factors. Therefore, caring for sleep is a powerful preventive measure to protect heart health and ensure more efficient and resilient cardiovascular function throughout life.

Metabolism, the complex process that converts food into energy, is another system vitally dependent on adequate sleep. As mentioned, hormonal dysregulation caused by sleep deprivation directly affects appetite control and can lead to weight gain. Furthermore, lack of sleep impacts how the body processes glucose, decreasing insulin sensitivity. This means cells have difficulty absorbing glucose from the blood, which can lead to high blood sugar levels and significantly increase the risk of developing type 2 diabetes. Maintaining a regular and sufficient sleep pattern helps regulate energy metabolism, contributes to a healthy body weight, and protects against metabolic disorders that can have serious long-term consequences.

The relationship between sleep, memory, and cognition is undeniable. As explored earlier, sleep, especially stages N3 and REM, is crucial for memory consolidation, the process by which newly acquired information is stabilized and integrated into existing knowledge. Sleep deprivation impairs not only the ability to form new memories but also affects other essential cognitive functions such as attention, concentration, logical reasoning, decision-making, and problem-solving. A tired mind becomes less efficient, slower, and more prone to errors. Investing in quality sleep is investing directly in mental clarity, learning capacity, and overall intellectual performance—indispensable tools for navigating the complexity of modern life.

Finally, mental health finds one of its most important regulators in sleep. The link between sleep disorders and mental health problems, such as depression and anxiety, is bidirectional and well-established. Insomnia and other sleep problems are common symptoms in depressive and anxious states, but sleep deprivation can also act as a trigger or aggravating factor for these conditions. REM sleep, in particular, plays a vital role in emotional processing and mood regulation. When we don't sleep enough or the quality of sleep is poor, our ability to cope with stress decreases, emotional reactivity increases, and the overall perspective can become more negative. Prioritizing sleep is a fundamental strategy to promote emotional stability, increase psychological resilience, and support the treatment of mental health conditions.

It becomes evident, therefore, that sleep is not a luxury but a transversal biological necessity that permeates and sustains all aspects of our health. Viewing it as such is an essential paradigm shift for anyone seeking not just to remedy problems but to cultivate a state of deep and lasting well-being. The scientific evidence linking good sleep to the prevention of chronic diseases, improved cognitive function, weight regulation, and mood stability is robust and growing.

Caring for sleep is caring for the body and mind in an integrated way. It's recognizing that, in the restorative silence of the night, we lay the foundations for more vibrant, healthy, and fulfilling days.

Given the many connections between sleep and the main axes of human health, its centrality becomes increasingly difficult to ignore. Nightly rest, contrary to what is still preached in discourses of productivity at all costs, is a sophisticated mechanism of self-preservation. It is a profoundly intelligent process where each physiological system, by tuning into the body's natural rhythms, finds ideal conditions to regenerate. Thus, sleep not only accompanies our living: it qualifies it, expands its possibilities, and sustains its continuity with balance and harmony. When well cared for, it transforms into a kind of silent medicine, acting without fanfare but with surprising effectiveness.

This awareness invites us to a practical and cultural change. In a world that constantly challenges our limits with artificial lights, long workdays, and incessant stimuli, protecting sleep is almost an act of resistance. It means choosing to stop where everything conspires towards movement. It also means recognizing that self-care is not indulgence, but responsibility. The quality of our sleep begins long before we lie down: in dietary choices, established schedules, stress management, and the routines we cultivate. Building this care does not require perfection, but consistency and presence—a real commitment to one's own well-being.

Sleeping well doesn't solve all health challenges, but it makes each one lighter to face. When we wake up truly restored, we face life with more clarity, strength, and emotional stability. More than just a habit, sleep reveals itself as a sophisticated tool for preserving life, an ancestral wisdom inscribed in every cell. Cultivating this bond is honoring the wholeness of being—body, mind, and spirit in silent communion each night. And it is in this daily, often invisible gesture, that we begin to build a health measured not just by the absence of disease, but by the full presence of vitality.

Chapter 4
Modern Barriers

Having recognized the invaluable worth of sleep, understood its cyclical architecture, and established its vital connection to integral health, a natural question arises: why, despite all this importance, do so many of us struggle to achieve truly restorative rest? The answer, in large part, lies in the complex and sometimes insidious barriers that modern life has erected between us and the innate ability to sleep well. We are immersed in an environment and a rhythm that often conspire against our biological clocks, creating a scenario where quality sleep becomes a challenge rather than a natural state. Identifying these contemporary villains of rest is a crucial step, a turning point that invites us to reflect on our own habits and the world around us, preparing the ground for conscious changes and the reclaiming of peaceful nights.

One of the most omnipresent barriers is, paradoxically, light. Our ancestors lived in sync with the natural cycles of light and darkness, with the sun dictating periods of activity and the night inviting withdrawal. The invention of artificial light, though a civilizational milestone, drastically altered this relationship. Today, we are exposed to constant illumination that extends far beyond sunset, coming from lamps, televisions, computers, tablets, and smartphones. This nighttime exposure to light, especially the blue light emitted by electronic devices, sends confusing signals to our brain. The suprachiasmatic nucleus, our central biological clock, interprets this light as if it were still daytime, suppressing the production of melatonin, the essential hormone that signals the body it's time to sleep. The result is difficulty falling asleep, shallower sleep, and a misaligned circadian cycle. We are, in a way, tricking our own bodies, keeping them in a state of alertness when they should be preparing for rest.

Hyperconnectivity and excessive screen use are extensions of this light barrier, but they bring additional layers of disruption. The need or desire to be constantly online, responding to messages, checking social media, or consuming information until the last moments before bed, keeps the mind in a state of agitation. The incessant flow of stimuli, notifications, and the very interactive nature of these technologies activate brain areas associated with attention and information processing, exactly the opposite of what we need to relax and fall asleep. Beyond the impact of blue light, the content consumed – whether it's work, worrying news, or exciting entertainment – can generate anxiety, stress, or simply keep the brain "switched on," making the smooth transition to sleep difficult. The habit of taking the smartphone to bed has become one of the biggest saboteurs of rest today.

Constant stress is another giant haunting our nights. Modern life, with its professional, financial, social, and family pressures, often places us in a state of chronic alert. The sympathetic nervous system, responsible for the "fight or flight" response, remains activated for longer than it should, releasing hormones like cortisol and adrenaline. These hormones, while useful in situations of real danger, are enemies of sleep when present in excess at the end of the day. They increase heart rate, blood pressure, and mental activity, making it almost impossible to relax and surrender to rest. The mind, caught in a cycle of worries, planning, or rumination, refuses to switch off. Stress not only makes it difficult to fall asleep but can also cause frequent nighttime awakenings, fragmenting sleep and compromising its restorative quality.

Our eating habits also play a significant role. Heavy, fatty, or very spicy meals close to bedtime can cause digestive discomfort, heartburn, or indigestion, hindering relaxation. The consumption of stimulants like caffeine, present not only in coffee but also in teas, sodas, and chocolates, can persist in the body for hours, blocking adenosine receptors – a substance that promotes sleepiness – and keeping us alert. Alcohol, although it may initially induce drowsiness, disrupts sleep architecture later in the night, especially REM sleep, leading to fragmented and non-restorative rest. Excessive hydration before bed can also lead to interruptions for bathroom trips. Lack of attention to what and when we eat and drink can silently sabotage our efforts to sleep well.

The lack of a consistent routine is another barrier imposed by the modern lifestyle. Irregular work schedules, social commitments extending late into the night, or simply the tendency to drastically vary sleep and wake times between weekdays and weekends confuse our biological clock. The human body thrives on regularity. Having consistent times for sleeping and waking, even on Saturdays and Sundays, helps synchronize our circadian rhythm, making it easier to fall asleep at night and wake up feeling refreshed in the morning. The absence of this regularity creates a state similar to "social jet lag," where our internal clock is constantly trying to adjust to different time zones, resulting in daytime sleepiness, difficulty concentrating, and problems sleeping at night.

This chapter serves as an invitation to self-observation. Which of these barriers resonate most strongly with your own experience? How does artificial light permeate your nights? What role do screens play in your pre-sleep routine? In what ways does stress manifest in your ability to relax? How might your eating habits and the regularity (or lack thereof) of your schedules be impacting your rest? Reflecting on these questions is not an exercise in guilt, but in awareness. It's the first step in recognizing that many of our sleep challenges are not personal failures, but understandable responses to an environment that often does not favor rest.

By understanding how these external and internal factors interfere with the delicate brain mechanisms regulating sleep, especially melatonin production, we gain power. From this new awareness, we are called to act intentionally. Breaking the automatic cycles that fuel sleep deprivation requires more than willpower: it demands sensitivity to identify what in our daily lives can be softened or reoriented. This sometimes means giving up certain immediate comforts – like one last look at social media or one more episode of that engaging series – in the name of deeper, lasting well-being. It also means rescuing the value of simple rituals: a darkened environment, a slower pace in the hours leading up to sleep, time reserved for quieting the body and mind. Small conscious choices, repeated consistently, can have a profound impact on the quality of rest and, consequently, on the quality of life as a whole.

By recognizing these barriers as constructions of modernity – and not as immutable aspects of existence – we open space for real transformations. The world around us will hardly slow down, but we can create havens of care within our routine, anchor points that reconnect us to the natural cycle of rest and wakefulness. Reconfiguring this bond with sleep is, in fact, an exercise in reconnecting with our own internal rhythms. It's a gesture of respect for this biological intelligence that, even amidst the chaotic demands of contemporary life, continues to ask for space to restore, integrate, and heal. When we heed this request, we rediscover sleep not as something to be conquered, but as a state to which we return, by choice and by merit. And it is in this return that we find what we often lack: the feeling of full repose, of restored presence, of body and mind in alliance. Identifying modern barriers to sleep is not an act of lament, but an invitation to autonomy. It's understanding that, even in the face of external pressures, we have room to act. We can choose, every day, to walk towards a more integral and respected sleep. Because, by caring for sleep, we care for the most silent – and therefore most essential – part of ourselves.

Chapter 5
Personal Diagnosis

The journey towards restorative sleep becomes clearer when we move from a general understanding of mechanisms and modern barriers to a more intimate and personalized look at our own experience. After identifying the potential villains lurking in our nights, the time comes to shine a light on our individual habits, routines, and perceptions. This chapter is an invitation to an honest and detailed self-assessment, a deep dive into the particularities that define our unique relationship with rest. This isn't about seeking a formal clinical diagnosis, but about cultivating keen self-awareness capable of revealing the patterns, difficulties, and specific needs shaping our nights. Taking on the role of investigator of one's own life is essential, because only from this personal clarity can we chart a path of truly effective and meaningful transformation, becoming active agents of our own healing and well-being.

Initiating this personal diagnosis requires, first and foremost, a willingness for attentive and non-judgmental observation. Let's start with the basics: schedules. What is, truly, your sleep pattern? Try to record, for a period of one or two weeks, the time you usually go to bed and the time you actually believe you fell asleep. Also, note the time you wake up in the morning and the time you get out of bed. Observe if there are significant variations in these times between weekdays and weekends. This simple data collection can reveal significant inconsistencies, the "social jet lag" mentioned earlier, or perhaps a discrepancy between time spent in bed and actual sleep time. Is there regularity, or does chaos prevail? At what time does your body naturally seem to feel sleepy, and at what time does it wake up spontaneously, if given the chance?

The perceived quality of rest is another pillar of this self-assessment. Upon waking, how do you feel? Refreshed, willing, and ready for the day, or still tired, groggy, and struggling to emerge from the sleep fog? This morning sensation is a valuable indicator of the efficiency of your nightly rest. Try to quantify this feeling, perhaps on a scale of 1 to 5, where 1 represents feeling exhausted and 5 fully restored. Observe how this perception varies day after day. Are there patterns? Days after specific nights where you feel better or worse? Also note the occurrence of morning headaches, dry mouth, or sore throat, which might indicate issues like bruxism or sleep-disordered breathing, although confirmation requires professional evaluation.

Nighttime awakenings deserve special attention. It's common to wake up briefly during the night, often without even remembering it in the morning. However, frequent, prolonged awakenings, or those that make it difficult to return to sleep, are warning signs. How many times do you estimate you wake up during the night? Do you remember the reason – to use the bathroom, because of noise, anxiety, or for no apparent reason? How long does it take to fall back asleep after these awakenings? Sleep fragmentation, even if the total time in bed is long, prevents proper progression through the NREM-REM cycles, severely compromising the restorative function of rest. Recording the frequency and nature of these awakenings helps identify potential triggers and assess the true depth of your sleep.

The bedroom environment, our sanctuary of rest, cannot be neglected in this investigation. Critically observe the space where you sleep. Is it dark enough? Small cracks of external light or the glow of electronic devices can interfere with melatonin production. Is it quiet? Noise from the street, neighbors, or even within the house can cause micro-arousals that fragment sleep. Is the temperature pleasant? Excessive heat or cold makes it difficult to fall asleep and maintain sleep. Do your mattress and pillows offer adequate comfort and support? An uncomfortable environment sends warning signals to the body, hindering deep relaxation. Evaluate each of these elements – light, sound, temperature, comfort – and reflect on how they might be contributing, positively or negatively, to the quality of your nights.

Finally, extend your observation beyond the night and assess your energy levels throughout the day. Do you feel alert and willing most of the day, or do you experience sharp drops in energy, excessive sleepiness, or difficulty concentrating, especially in the afternoon? The frequent need for naps or high caffeine consumption to stay awake can be indicators of insufficient or poor-quality nighttime sleep. Also, observe your general mood, patience, and ability to cope with daily stress. As we've seen, sleep directly impacts our emotional balance. Significant mood swings or constant irritability may be related to poorly slept nights. Connecting daytime sensations with nighttime sleep quality reinforces the understanding of the interdependence between rest and wakefulness.

This process of personal diagnosis, which can be aided by keeping a detailed sleep diary (something we will explore further later), is fundamentally an exercise in self-knowledge. There are no right or wrong answers, only your individual truth emerging through careful observation. By gathering this information – about your schedules, perceived sleep quality, awakenings, bedroom environment, and your daytime energy levels and mood – you begin to paint a clearer picture of your current situation. Understanding your particular difficulties is the essential step that allows you to tailor future techniques and strategies to your real needs. Instead of following generic recipes, you will be building a personalized path.

As you assemble this mosaic of information about yourself, what emerges is much more than a portrait of sleep: it's a mirror of your own routine, the impacts of the external world on your body, and the way you listen – or don't – to yourself daily. This active listening, free from excessive self-criticism, reveals important nuances often overlooked in the daily rush. A recurring awakening at three in the morning, persistent drowsiness after lunch, or a more unstable emotional state in certain weeks are not random: they are messages from the body asking for attention. The sleep diary, in this sense, acts as a kind of translator between what we feel and what we actually experience in our sleep patterns. It transforms subjective sensations into valuable data, making visible what was previously hidden in uncertainty.

This investigative journey also invites us to recognize the individuality of sleep. What works for one person may not work for another. Some benefit from nighttime meditations, while others find tranquility in light reading or the simple ritual of preparing warm tea. Some need absolute silence, while others sleep better with white noise in the background. The most important thing is to understand that the answer isn't out there, in ready-made formulas or wellness trends, but within, in the sincere listening to one's own body and in the responses that emerge from the continuous practice of self-observation. When we become experts on ourselves, we also become more compassionate, more patient, and better prepared to adjust routes gently and intentionally.

At the end of this process, sleep ceases to be an enigma disconnected from the rest of life and becomes part of a broader system of choices, sensations, and needs. The personal diagnosis is not an endpoint, but a lucid starting point. With this map in hand, the path towards restorative sleep becomes less nebulous and more accessible. The transformation begins, then, with a simple but powerful gesture: looking at oneself with curiosity, courage, and the genuine desire to care. Because sleeping well is not just a health goal – it's a return to the essence of living with presence, balance, and self-respect.

Chapter 6
Concept of Sanctuary

The path to deep, restorative sleep is not limited to our habits and internal biology; it extends to the physical space where rest occurs. The bedroom, often treated as just another room in the house, holds transformative potential when viewed through a new lens: that of a true sanctuary dedicated to repose. This concept goes far beyond mere decoration or organization. It involves intentionally cultivating an environment that invites peace, comfort, and a necessary detachment from the pressures and stimuli of the outside world. The idea of a sanctuary evokes a sacred, safe, and tranquil place, and it is precisely this atmosphere we seek to create in the space where we surrender to the vulnerability and renewal of sleep. Recognizing the power of the physical environment over our mental and emotional state is fundamental, as deep rest begins long before we close our eyes; it begins when the space itself whispers to us that it's time to slow down, withdraw, and trust.

Transforming the bedroom into a sleep sanctuary involves careful attention to sensory details, starting with lighting. As we've seen, light has a direct impact on regulating our circadian cycle. While access to natural light during the day is beneficial, as night approaches, the intensity and tone of light in the bedroom should change. Opting for soft, warm, indirect lighting in the hours leading up to sleep helps signal to the brain that the day is ending. Lamps with low-wattage bulbs and yellow or amber tones are preferable to bright white ceiling lights. Using dimmers to control light intensity allows for environmental adjustments as needed. Total darkness during sleep is ideal for maximum melatonin production, so blackout curtains or sleep masks can be valuable allies in blocking any residual external or internal light, creating a protective cocoon.

Organization and the absence of visual clutter are other essential pillars in building this sanctuary. A cluttered room, with piles of clothes, work papers, or objects unrelated to rest, acts as constant visual noise, conveying a sense of pending tasks and mental chaos. The external environment reflects and influences our internal state. A clean, organized, minimalist space, where every object has its place and purpose, promotes a sense of calm, clarity, and control. It's important to remove anything from the bedroom that reminds you of work, stress, or excessive stimulation. Turning off or, ideally, removing electronic devices like televisions, computers, and even smartphones significantly contributes to creating a distraction-free zone dedicated exclusively to rest and intimacy. Visual simplicity calms the mind and facilitates the process of disengagement.

Air quality and proper ventilation are also crucial. A stuffy room or one with unpleasant odors hinders relaxation. Ensuring good air circulation, either by opening windows during the day or using an air purifier, contributes to a fresher, cleaner, and more pleasant environment. The temperature, as mentioned in the self-assessment, should be maintained at a slightly cooler level, considered ideal by most experts for promoting quality sleep, generally between 18 and 21 degrees Celsius (64 to 70 degrees Fahrenheit). The body needs to lower its core temperature to initiate and maintain sleep, and a cool environment facilitates this natural process. Adjusting the thermostat, using season-appropriate bedding, or silent fans can make a significant difference in thermal comfort.

The textures of the materials we come into contact with in the bedroom also influence our perception of comfort and welcome. Choosing soft, breathable sheets made from natural fibers like cotton or linen can transform the experience of lying down. Blankets and duvets that offer the right weight and warmth, without causing overheating, contribute to a feeling of security and coziness. Soft rugs underfoot, curtains with a nice drape, and even the texture of the walls can add layers of sensory comfort to the environment. Paying attention to these tactile details helps create a space that embraces us and invites deep relaxation, where the body feels safe and nurtured.

Aromatherapy can be a powerful tool to complement the sanctuary's atmosphere. Certain scents have proven abilities to calm the nervous system and induce relaxation. Essential oils like lavender, chamomile, sandalwood, or marjoram can be used in electric diffusers, room sprays, or applied to pulse points (diluted in carrier oil) before sleep. The sense of smell has a direct connection to the limbic system, the area of the brain associated with emotions and memory, making aromas a quick and effective way to influence our state of mind. Choosing a scent that personally brings you feelings of calm and well-being can add a final, deeply personal touch to your sleep sanctuary.

Finally, creating a sound sanctuary is essential, especially in noisy urban environments. The goal is to minimize disruptive sounds that can fragment sleep. In addition to windows with good sound insulation, using earplugs or white noise generators can be very effective. White noise, a constant sound that masks other sound frequencies, can muffle sudden noises and create a stable, calming auditory background, making it easier to fall asleep and maintain sleep. The important thing is to find what works best to create a bubble of auditory tranquility.

Reflecting on your own bedroom in light of these elements is a revealing exercise. How does your current space compare to this vision of a sanctuary? What small or large changes could be implemented to make it more welcoming, peaceful, and conducive to rest? Transforming the bedroom into a sanctuary doesn't require large investments, but rather intention and care. It's an ongoing process of adjustment and refinement, guided by the perception of how the physical environment directly impacts our ability to relax the mind and surrender the body to repose.

Building this sleep sanctuary is, in essence, an act of conscious self-care. Each element, from the fabric touching the skin to the aroma filling the air, conveys a silent message of welcome and presence. And it's in this attention to seemingly simple details that the environment's transformative power lies. By shaping a space that respects the body's rhythms and aligns with the spirit's needs, we are, in fact, cultivating an intimate pact with ourselves: to honor rest as an essential part of life. The bedroom ceases to be just a backdrop for the end of the day and becomes a refuge where time slows down, and the body finds permission to simply be.

It's important to remember that this process of sanctification doesn't demand perfection, but sensitivity. Small rituals, like dimming the lights more slowly, making the bed meticulously, or playing soft music in the background, act as symbolic gestures communicating to the unconscious that the time for withdrawal has arrived. By making the space an extension of our values of well-being and serenity, we create a virtuous cycle: the more the environment favors rest, the more the body learns to relax in that place, and the deeper and more restorative sleep becomes. Thus, the bedroom also transforms into an emotional anchor, a point of stability amidst the uncertainties of daily life. In this carefully woven shelter of intentions and choices, sleep ceases to be just a physiological function and takes on the role of a restorative rite. The sleep sanctuary is not an unattainable ideal, but a tangible expression of personal care, capable of sustaining more serene nights and, consequently, more lucid and vigorous days. In this sacred space, every gesture – no matter how small it seems – contributes to building an environment where silence is welcome, darkness is gentle, and repose becomes an invitation to daily healing.

Chapter 7
Sleep Hygiene

Building a physical sanctuary for rest, as discussed in the previous chapter, establishes a fundamental foundation for quieter nights. However, the journey to truly restorative sleep also involves refining our daily habits and routines. This is where the concept of "sleep hygiene" comes in—a term that might sound clinical, but essentially refers to a set of practices and behaviors we can adopt during the day, and especially in the hours leading up to bedtime, to naturally promote better quality sleep. It involves recognizing that small daily actions, often overlooked, have a cumulative and significant impact on our ability to fall asleep, stay asleep, and wake up feeling restored. Sleep hygiene isn't a magic formula to cure complex sleep disorders overnight, but rather the conscious construction of a solid foundation for well-being, an invitation to integrate simple and accessible practices that prepare the ground for sleep to flourish.

One of the most important pillars of sleep hygiene is regularity. Our bodies operate on a circadian rhythm, an internal biological clock that regulates sleep-wake cycles, among other functions. This clock thrives on consistency. Establishing regular times for going to bed and waking up, even on weekends or days off, is one of the most effective measures to synchronize our internal rhythm. Abrupt variations in these times confuse the brain, making both falling asleep and waking up more difficult. Try to set a sleep window that allows you to get the recommended amount of hours for your age group and strive to maintain it as consistently as possible. This regularity helps anchor the sleep-wake cycle, strengthening the natural signals of sleepiness at night and alertness in the morning. It may require discipline initially, but the benefits in terms of sleep quality and stable daytime energy are remarkable.

Exposure to natural light, especially in the morning, is another fundamental practice. Morning sunlight acts as a powerful synchronizer for our biological clock, signaling to the body that the day has begun and helping suppress residual nighttime melatonin. Try to spend a few minutes outdoors shortly after waking, whether having coffee on the balcony, walking to work, or simply opening the windows wide to let the light in. This morning exposure not only helps you wake up and improve your mood but also helps regulate melatonin production later, making it easier to fall asleep at the right time. Conversely, it's crucial to manage light exposure at night, as previously discussed. Reducing the intensity of home lighting and, crucially, avoiding the blue light emitted by screens of smartphones, tablets, and computers in the two to three hours before bed is essential. If use is unavoidable, consider using blue light filters or specific glasses.

What we do in the hours leading up to sleep directly impacts our ability to relax. Creating a "wind-down" period is vital. Avoid stimulating activities, both physically and mentally. Intense physical exercise should be avoided close to bedtime, although light activities like gentle stretching can be beneficial. Heated discussions, planning complex tasks, or consuming disturbing news can activate the mind and generate anxiety, hindering disengagement. Instead, reserve this time for relaxing activities that signal to your body and mind it's time to prepare for rest.

Ritualizing sleep, meaning creating a sequence of calming actions performed every night in the same order, can be extremely effective. This pre-sleep routine is highly personal but might include elements like taking a warm bath, which helps relax tense muscles and induces a slight drop in body temperature favorable for sleep; reading a physical book under soft light (avoiding overly stimulating reads); listening to calm music or a relaxing podcast; practicing deep breathing techniques or meditation for a few minutes; or writing in a journal to release worries and thoughts from the day. The key is consistency. Over time, these rituals become conditioned triggers, sending clear signals to the brain that sleep is approaching, facilitating the transition from wakefulness to rest.

Diet and hydration are also part of sleep hygiene. Avoiding heavy, fatty, or very spicy meals within three hours of bedtime prevents digestive discomfort. Opt for a lighter dinner and, if hunger strikes later, choose a small, easily digestible snack like a banana or a handful of almonds. Limiting fluid intake close to bedtime can reduce the need for nighttime bathroom trips. It's essential to avoid caffeine for at least six hours before bed and moderate or avoid alcohol consumption, especially at night, due to its disruptive effects on sleep architecture.

It's important to realize that sleep hygiene isn't a rigid list of rules to be followed perfectly, but rather a set of guidelines to be adapted to your reality and individual needs. The goal isn't to add more stress to your routine, but to identify and modify habits that might be harming your rest without you realizing it. Start by implementing one or two changes that seem most accessible and observe the results. Gradually integrate other practices as you feel comfortable. Consistency is more important than perfection.

By adopting these practices, you are building, day by day, a more solid foundation for quality sleep. Sleep hygiene works as preventive care, helping optimize the body's natural processes and creating the ideal conditions for rest to occur more efficiently and restoratively. It's not just about solving insomnia problems, but about cultivating a lifestyle that respects and actively supports the vital need to sleep well.

Just as important as adopting these practices is developing greater sensitivity to your own internal signals. The body constantly sends messages about its needs, and learning to listen attentively is an essential part of sleep hygiene. Signs of drowsiness, irritability, difficulty concentrating, or energy fluctuations throughout the day can indicate a misalignment between habits and the body's natural rhythm. Being aware of these signs allows for more precise adjustments to behaviors preceding sleep, promoting subtle yet effective interventions, such as starting the nightly ritual earlier or rethinking the use of electronic devices. This type of active listening transforms the sleep routine into a practice of continuous self-awareness and care.

Furthermore, it's crucial to consider the impact of lifestyle as a whole on sleep quality. Factors such as chronic stress levels, excessive responsibilities, or even the lack of leisure time and emotional connection during the day can directly affect nights. Sleep hygiene, therefore, is not isolated from other dimensions of well-being. It is strengthened when integrated into a broader approach to balance: setting aside time for genuine breaks, cultivating healthy relationships, maintaining mindful eating habits, and seeking regular physical activity. Sleep doesn't just begin at dusk; it is prepared throughout the day with choices that respect the rhythm of life and the body's limits.

With this more holistic perspective, sleep hygiene ceases to be a mere functional strategy and takes a leading role in maintaining overall health. Sleeping well is not a luxury; it's a physiological and emotional necessity—and caring for sleep is, ultimately, caring for life itself. By persisting in these practices with kindness and consistency, you will not only promote quieter nights but also build a more harmonious relationship with yourself, where rest and vitality walk side by side.

Chapter 8
Limiting Beliefs

The journey to reclaiming healthy, restorative sleep moves beyond environmental barriers and daily habits, entering a subtler yet equally powerful territory: the realm of our beliefs. Often, the greatest resistance to rest lies not in external factors, but in deeply ingrained ideas, both cultural and personal, that shape our perception and relationship with the act of sleeping. These limiting beliefs, frequently operating at an unconscious level, can sabotage our best efforts to implement sleep hygiene practices or create an environment conducive to repose. Identifying, questioning, and ultimately deconstructing these notions is a fundamental step to clearing the path and allowing a new mindset to flourish – one that recognizes sleep not as a burden or a waste of time, but as a sacred act of self-care, deservingness, and profound self-love.

One of the most pervasive beliefs in contemporary society links sleep to unproductivity or even laziness. In a culture that glorifies constant hustle, being "always busy," and the ability to operate on little sleep, rest is often relegated to the background, seen as a dispensable luxury or a necessary evil that steals precious hours from work, study, or leisure. Phrases like "sleep is for the weak" or "I'll sleep when I'm dead" echo this toxic mentality, which equates human value with the capacity for incessant production. We internalize this pressure and start feeling guilty for needing to rest, pushing our limits and ignoring the body's exhaustion signals in the name of supposed efficiency. This belief ignores the vast scientific evidence demonstrating the exact opposite: adequate sleep is a fundamental pillar of sustainable productivity, creativity, mental clarity, and optimal performance in any area of life. Sacrificing sleep for productivity is, in the long run, shooting oneself in the foot.

This "productivity at all costs" mentality often leads us to view sleep as an enemy to be conquered or controlled, rather than an ally to be cultivated. We try to "cheat" sleep with caffeine, poorly planned strategic naps, or simply resisting drowsiness to the limit. When insomnia arises, frustration and anxiety set in, creating a vicious cycle where the fear of not being able to sleep becomes, itself, an obstacle to sleep. The underlying belief is that we should be able to "switch off" our minds on command, like a machine, and the inability to do so is seen as a personal failure. This adversarial approach ignores the delicate and responsive nature of our nervous system, which needs safety, relaxation, and permission to surrender to rest, not struggle or forced control.

Beyond cultural influences, we also carry our own personal beliefs, shaped by past experiences, family dynamics, or even trauma. For some people, night might be associated with feelings of loneliness, fear, or vulnerability, especially if there were childhood experiences of fear of the dark, recurring nightmares, or an insecure family environment at night. The act of falling asleep, which involves a loss of control and consciousness, can be unconsciously perceived as threatening. In other cases, bedtime might have been associated with family conflicts, arguments, or tensions, creating an internal resistance to going to bed. Beliefs like "I don't deserve to rest" or "I need to be always alert" may have roots in feelings of guilt, low self-esteem, or past experiences where constant vigilance was necessary for self-preservation. Recognizing these connections, sometimes painful, is an important step in understanding deeper resistances to sleep.

Habits inherited or learned in childhood can also perpetuate limiting beliefs. If we grew up in an environment where adults slept little, valued night work, or expressed negative views about sleep, it's likely we internalized these attitudes without questioning them. The way our parents or caregivers handled our own childhood sleep – whether there was excessive rigidity, lack of routine, or anxiety around falling asleep – can also leave lasting marks on our relationship with rest in adulthood. We become adults who replicate old patterns, often unaware of their origin or current impact.

Deconstructing these limiting beliefs requires conscious work of mental reprogramming. The first step is identification: what thoughts or feelings arise when you think about sleeping, resting, or taking time for yourself? Do you feel guilty, anxious, impatient? Do you believe sleeping less makes you stronger or more dedicated? Write down these ideas and question their validity. Are they really yours, or were they absorbed from the external environment? Are they based on facts or cultural pressures? Confronting these beliefs with the reality of sleep benefits and your own bodily needs is essential.

The next step is to actively replace limiting beliefs with affirmations and perspectives that honor the value of rest. Start cultivating the idea that sleeping well is not a luxury, but a fundamental right and an act of intelligence. See sleep as an investment in your health, well-being, and ability to live fully. Affirm to yourself that you deserve to rest, that your body needs this time to recover, and that caring for your sleep is an expression of self-love. Reframe rest not as lost time, but as gained vitality, clarity, and resilience. Celebrate well-slept nights as important achievements for your overall health.

This reprogramming doesn't happen overnight. It requires constant vigilance over automatic thoughts and a conscious effort to choose a new narrative. It might involve forgiving yourself for neglecting sleep in the past and committing to a different future. In some cases, especially when deep trauma or emotional issues are involved, seeking therapeutic support can be crucial to untangle these knots and build a safer, more peaceful relationship with the act of sleeping.

By challenging and transforming these limiting beliefs, we make space for a new relationship with sleep, one based on respect, permission, and understanding of its vital importance. We stop fighting against our need for rest and start welcoming it as an essential part of our humanity. The mindset shifts from sacrifice to self-care, from guilt to deservingness.

In this process of transformation, sleep comes to be understood not just as a physiological function, but as a symbolic space where the quality of the bond we maintain with ourselves is revealed. Abandoning beliefs that reinforce constant vigilance, control, and disregard for the body's needs requires courage, because it invites us into contact with vulnerabilities we have long sought to silence.

By revisiting memories, questioning inherited narratives, and offering ourselves new ways to signify rest, we undertake a healing movement that reverberates beyond well-slept nights—it also touches how we value ourselves, how we perceive ourselves as worthy of peace and relief.

This new mindset invites us to step beyond the technical and practical strategies that support sleep, diving into a more intimate plane where rest also becomes a process of reconciliation. Reconciling with our own fatigue, with the body's limits, with the natural need to pause. Each night we allow ourselves to rest without guilt, even amidst external or internal demands insisting on urgency, we reaffirm the right to exist with lightness.

Sleeping well, in this context, also becomes a political and existential gesture: refusing exhaustion as a way of life and choosing a gentler path, more attuned to the body's wisdom. Thus, by deactivating the beliefs that distanced us from sleep, we clear the way for a fuller, more integrated experience of rest. The night ceases to be a territory of struggle or punishment and transforms into a time of regeneration and care. Sleep, then, is no longer a challenge to be overcome, but a space that welcomes us—not as productive machines on pause, but as living beings who, by sleeping, reaffirm their connection to their own natural rhythm, to their own dignity. In this restorative silence, we rediscover not only rest, but something even deeper: the permission to be whole.

Chapter 9
Sleep in History

Our contemporary relationship with sleep, often marked by neglect, the fight against drowsiness, or the medicalization of insomnia, contrasts sharply with the view many ancient and traditional cultures held about this fundamental state of existence. By looking back at how different civilizations throughout history and around the world perceived and integrated rest into their lives, we discover a wealth of perspectives that can inspire us to reclaim a sense of reverence and connection with our own cycles of repose. Exploring sleep in history is not just an exercise in intellectual curiosity; it's an opportunity to reflect on how much our modern view, often purely mechanistic and focused on productivity, has drifted from a more natural, integrated, and even sacred understanding of the act of sleeping. This symbolic reclaiming can help us restore a more respectful and harmonious relationship with our own sleep, preparing the ground to welcome the practices and techniques to come.

In many ancient traditions, sleep was not seen as mere physiological shutdown but as a portal to other dimensions of reality, a time of deep connection with the divine, with ancestors, or with the deeper layers of one's own psyche. In ancient Egypt, for example, dreams were considered messages from the gods, and there were temples dedicated to dream incubation, where people slept hoping to receive divine guidance or healing for their ailments. Dream interpretation was a valued art, and it was believed that the dream world offered precious insights for waking life. This view imbues sleep with a dimension of mystery and revealing potential that we rarely consider today.

In ancient Greece, Hypnos, the god of sleep, was an important deity, twin brother of Thanatos (Death) and son of Nyx (Night). Sleep was personified and respected, associated with calm and restorative rest. Temples dedicated to Asclepius, the god of healing, also practiced dream incubation (enkoimesis), where the sick slept in sacred precincts hoping the god would appear in a dream to indicate a cure. This practice demonstrates a profound belief in the intrinsic therapeutic power of sleep and dreams, a wisdom that modern medicine is beginning to rediscover by investigating the processes of physical and emotional repair that occur during rest.

Many indigenous cultures around the world maintain views of sleep and dreams as integral parts of spiritual and community life. For various Native American peoples, dreams are essential sources of guidance, shamanic knowledge, and connection with the spiritual world. Nightly rituals, storytelling before bed, and community sharing of dreams in the morning were common practices, reinforcing the idea that sleep is a space for vital learning and communication. Similarly, in many African traditions, sleep is the time when the soul can travel, meet ancestral spirits, and receive important messages for the individual and the community. Respect for elders, who often need more rest, and the integration of the natural rhythm of day and night into daily life reflect a harmony with natural cycles that we have often lost.

In Asian cultures, we also find a valuation of rest and specific practices related to sleep. In traditional Chinese medicine, sleep is considered essential for balancing Yin and Yang and for the proper circulation of Qi (vital energy). Sleep disturbances are seen as symptoms of deeper energy imbalances. Practices like meditation, Tai Chi, and acupuncture are often used to promote harmonious sleep. In Japan, although modern culture also faces challenges with sleep deprivation, there is the cultural practice of "inemuri," meaning "being present while sleeping" – the social acceptance of briefly dozing in public, such as on transport or in meetings, recognizing the body's natural need for rest without the stigma of laziness.

This integrated and often reverent view of sleep began to transform drastically with the advent of the Industrial Revolution in Europe and subsequently in other parts of the world. The invention of artificial lighting, as mentioned, allowed the workday to extend beyond the natural cycle of sunlight. Factories, with their rigid shifts and long hours of labor, began to dictate the rhythm of life, and sleep started to be seen as an obstacle to production. The need to synchronize workers with machine schedules led to a standardization of sleep patterns, often ignoring individual needs and biological rhythms. Time became rigidly measured and monetized, and the time dedicated to sleep began to be perceived as "unproductive." This utilitarian mentality gradually infiltrated the culture, stripping sleep of its intrinsic value and sacred dimension. Rest became secondary, something to be done only as strictly necessary to keep the human machine running.

The pressure for productivity, the rise of capitalism, and the valuation of individualism contributed to sleep being increasingly neglected, associated with weakness or lack of ambition. We lost connection with nightly rituals, with observing nature's cycles, and with listening to our own body's needs. The night, once a time of mystery, withdrawal, and connection, often became just an interval to be overcome as quickly as possible to resume the day's incessant activity.

Reflecting on this historical trajectory invites us to question the normality of our current relationship with sleep. Is the modern view, focused solely on physiological aspects and often marked by struggle and anxiety, the only possible way to face rest? By recalling how other cultures valued sleep as a time for healing, revelation, and spiritual connection, we can begin to reclaim a sense of purpose and meaning for our own nights. It's not about literally replicating ancient practices, but about being inspired by their essence: respect for natural rhythm, valuation of withdrawal, openness to mystery, and understanding sleep as an integral and vital part of the human experience.

This symbolic reclaiming has the power to transform our attitude towards sleep. Instead of seeing it as an obligation or a problem to be solved, we can begin to view it as a gift, a daily opportunity for physical, mental, emotional, and perhaps even spiritual renewal. We can cultivate the intention to make our sleep a sacred time, a sanctuary not only physical but also mental. This shift in perspective, nurtured by the wisdom of the past, can be a powerful catalyst for adopting, with more meaning and commitment, the practices that promote deep and restorative rest.

Reconnecting with the symbolic and ancestral value of sleep invites us to slow down not just the body, but also the soul. Remembering that entire civilizations once celebrated rest as a time for healing and inner listening encourages us to rethink our rush to "solve" sleep with quick fixes and isolated techniques. True transformation lies in how we choose to relate to the night, to silence, and to the invisible spaces it opens.

Perhaps it is in this recognition—that sleeping is not erasing oneself, but rather returning to a part of us that the day keeps in suspension—that we can reverse the logic of deprivation and embrace sleep as a fertile time of reunion. This symbolic valuation, however, need not contradict the advances of modern science but can coexist with them in a complementary way.

If, on one hand, we better understand the neurochemical and physiological processes that occur during sleep, on the other, we can recover the sensitivity that ancient traditions had in intuiting, without devices or measurements, that there was something sacred and transformative there.

Integrating these dimensions—technical knowledge and symbolic knowledge—is an essential step in reclaiming sleep as a full and unfragmented well-being. This implies not only creating ideal routines or environments but also restoring an attitude of reverence before the very need to rest, like honoring an essential part of life.

By understanding that neglecting sleep is ultimately neglecting existence itself in its totality, we make space for a new pact with the night. Sleeping, thus, becomes an act of trust: trusting that the world can go on while we rest, that we don't need to control everything all the time, that there is wisdom in stopping. Inspired by centuries of traditions that knew how to see in sleep a bridge to something greater, we can choose not just to sleep more, but to sleep with more presence, more surrender, and more meaning. And it is in this silent gesture of closing our eyes with respect that, perhaps, we rediscover the sleep that the modern world taught us to fear or despise.

Chapter 10
Introduction to Sleep Tourism

As our understanding of the vital importance of sleep deepens and we recognize the barriers imposed by modern life, as well as the beliefs that limit us, an interesting and revealing movement emerges in the contemporary scene: so-called "sleep tourism." This concept, gaining strength in recent years, reflects a growing awareness of the need for quality rest and the desire to actively seek environments and experiences specifically designed to promote nocturnal restoration. Hotels, spas, retreats, and entire destinations are beginning to specialize in offering more than just a comfortable bed; they propose an immersion in practices and technologies aimed at reprogramming and optimizing visitors' sleep. Introducing this trend is not just presenting a new travel modality, but rather broadening our perspective on the possibilities of sleep care, showing that the quest for well-slept nights can even transform into a pleasurable, enriching, and profoundly transformative experience, whose principles can inspire changes even within our own homes.

Sleep tourism starts from the premise that the environment and routines during a trip can be powerful tools to break unsatisfactory sleep patterns and re-establish a healthier rhythm. Away from the pressures and stimuli of daily life, in a space carefully planned for relaxation, the traveler has the opportunity to disconnect from sources of stress and reconnect with themselves and their need for rest. These specialized places invest heavily in creating ideal conditions for repose. Rooms are designed to be true sanctuaries, with impeccable sound insulation to ensure silence, blackout curtains for total darkness, precise temperature control systems, and high-quality bedding, often with personalized options for pillows and mattresses adapting to individual preferences. Attention to sensory details is paramount, seeking to eliminate any element that could disturb the tranquility necessary to fall asleep and stay asleep.

Beyond the physical infrastructure, the differential of sleep tourism lies in the therapies and programs offered. Many of these establishments employ sleep specialists, therapists, or coaches who assist guests in diagnosing their challenges and developing personalized strategies. Guided meditation sessions specifically designed to induce relaxation before sleep, conscious breathing practices, restorative yoga, or gentle tai chi may be offered. Sound therapies, using white noise, nature sounds, or binaural beats, can be integrated into the room environment or offered in specific sessions to calm the mind and facilitate entry into deeper sleep states. Aromatherapy, with relaxing essential oils, is also frequently used in rooms or in nighttime spa treatments.

Technology also plays a role in some of these initiatives, with the use of non-invasive sleep monitoring devices providing feedback on the guest's rest quality, or smart beds that automatically adjust to optimize comfort and temperature. Some proposals even include "light hygiene" programs, with lighting systems simulating the natural sun cycle, helping regulate the visitor's biological clock, especially useful for those suffering from jet lag or working irregular shifts. The food offered in these places is also usually designed to favor sleep, with menus including ingredients known for their relaxing properties or that aid melatonin production, and with guidance on the best times for meals.

Exploring the possibilities offered by sleep tourism can be a powerful way to reconnect with one's own biological rhythm and intensively learn practices that favor rest. For those facing chronic sleep difficulties, spending a few days immersed in an environment fully dedicated to restoration can represent a significant turning point, offering not only temporary relief but also tools and insights to take home. It can be an opportunity to try different relaxation techniques, discover which environmental elements most positively impact one's own sleep, and receive professional guidance in a context free from usual distractions. This immersion acts as a "reset," allowing the body and mind to rediscover the sensation of deep rest and re-educate themselves on how to achieve it.

However, the inspiration provided by this concept is not limited to those who can or wish to travel to specialized destinations. The central principles and practices of sleep tourism can be adapted and applied in our own homes and routines. The idea of transforming the bedroom into a sanctuary, attention to lighting and noise, creating relaxing nightly rituals, exploring sound or aromatic therapies, choosing comfortable bedding – all this can be implemented in our daily lives, transforming our domestic environment into a space that actively promotes nocturnal well-being. We can be inspired by the offerings of these retreats to create our own "mini-sleep retreats" at home on weekends, dedicating intentional time to disconnection, relaxation, and applying learned techniques.

The emergence of sleep tourism as a trend reflects an important cultural shift: the growing recognition that sleep is not just a passive physiological need, but an active dimension of our health and well-being that deserves to be cultivated, cared for, and even celebrated. It shows that investing in one's own rest can be a legitimate and valuable form of leisure and self-investment. By broadening our view to include these possibilities, we realize that the quest for better sleep need not be an arduous and solitary journey; it can be faced as a pleasurable exploration, an adventure of self-knowledge, and an opportunity to experience new forms of relaxation and renewal. Whether through an actual trip or the inspired application of these concepts at home, the central idea is the same: honoring our sleep and recognizing its transformative power in our lives.

Incorporating sleep tourism into our lives ultimately represents an invitation to re-signify rest as an act of presence and celebration. The experience of withdrawing, even for a few days, from a routine that frequently suppresses silence, slow rhythm, and inner listening, reveals that sleep can be much more than an end of the day – it can be an experience of reconnecting with the essential. By experiencing an environment that values rest comprehensively, we are reminded that sleep is a state deserving space, care, and intention, not just a passive interval between obligations. This paradigm shift has the potential to generate profound reflections: seeing ourselves immersed in experiences that center rest, we learn that well-being begins with what we give ourselves permission to cease. Sleeping well becomes not just a functional goal, but a gesture of affection for oneself. In a world constantly pulling us outward, towards noise, towards excess, initiatives like sleep tourism signal the importance of returning to the body, to breath, and to the organic time of life. And the more we understand the value of this intentional pause, the more we open ourselves to reconstructing habits that support the continuity of this restorative state, even outside the specialized environment. Thus, sleep tourism presents itself not as an escape, but as a model of possibilities. It shows us that it is indeed possible to live more consciously regarding rest, and that this care need not be extraordinary to be transformative. The essential thing is the awakening to the need to nurture sleep with respect and creativity. From there, each night becomes a new opportunity to start anew — with less weight, more serenity, and the renewed disposition that only truly respected sleep can offer.

Chapter 11
The Nightly Ritualization

With the foundations of sleep knowledge firmly established – its importance, cycles, relationship with health, modern barriers, limiting beliefs, and historical and cultural perspectives – we now enter the territory of practical application. Part II of this book is dedicated to concrete techniques and strategies we can implement to actively cultivate deeper, more restorative rest. And the natural starting point for this practical transformation is the creation of a nightly ritual, a sequence of conscious and intentional actions performed consistently before sleep, with the purpose of signaling to the body and mind that the day is ending and it's time to prepare for repose.

Far from being a mystical or esoteric act, nightly ritualization is a powerful psychological and physiological tool, an effective way to condition our brain and nervous system to slow down, relax, and facilitate a smooth transition from wakefulness to sleep.

The core idea behind the nightly ritual is based on the power of habit and conditioning. Just as the sound of an alarm clock can put us on alert in the morning, a sequence of calming actions repeated every night creates a positive and predictable association with the act of sleeping. The brain learns to recognize these signals as precursors to sleep, beginning to release neurotransmitters and hormones that promote relaxation and drowsiness, such as adenosine and melatonin, while reducing the production of stimulating substances like cortisol. This conditioning process helps to "turn off" the day's agitated mind and prepare the body for rest more efficiently and naturally than simply turning off the light and hoping sleep will come. Consistent repetition is key; it transforms simple actions into powerful triggers for relaxation.

Building a personalized nightly ritual is a creative and individual process. There's no single formula that works for everyone, as what relaxes one person might stimulate another. The goal is to choose a set of activities that are genuinely calming and pleasant for you, and that can be performed consistently in the last hour, or the last 30 to 60 minutes, before your desired bedtime. It's important that these activities are carried out in a quiet environment, with soft light, and avoid exposure to bright screens or stimulating content. The beauty of the ritual lies in its simplicity and the intention we put into it: the intention to care for ourselves and honor our need for rest.

What activities can make up this ritual? The options are varied, and you can combine two or three that resonate most with you. A warm bath or foot soak, for example, are classic and effective practices. Warm water helps relax tense muscles, and upon getting out of the bath, the slight drop in body temperature signals to the brain that it's time to sleep. Adding Epsom salts, rich in magnesium (a mineral known for its relaxing properties), or a few drops of calming essential oils like lavender or chamomile can enhance the effect.

Aromatherapy, as mentioned, can be a powerful component of the ritual. Using a diffuser with relaxing essential oils in the bedroom while you prepare for sleep, or applying a pillow spray with a calming scent, can create an atmosphere conducive to sleep. Choose aromas that convey peace and tranquility to you, transforming the act of breathing into an invitation to relax.

Light reading is another excellent option for many. Choosing a physical book (avoiding screens) with content that isn't overly exciting or disturbing can help divert the mind from the day's worries and induce a state of calm. Reading poetry, quiet fiction, inspirational texts, or spiritual material can be a pleasant way to slow down mental activity before sleep.

Listening to calm music, nature sounds, relaxing podcasts, or guided meditations can also be part of your ritual. Music has a direct impact on our emotional and physiological state, and choosing soft, instrumental melodies or tracks with specific frequencies can help reduce heart rate and induce slower brain waves associated with relaxation and the initial stages of sleep.

Mindfulness and gratitude practices are valuable tools for calming the mind. Dedicating a few minutes to practice conscious breathing, focusing on the sensation of air entering and leaving the body, helps anchor the mind in the present and reduce rumination. Writing in a gratitude journal, noting three things you were grateful for that day, can shift the mental focus from what's lacking or worrying to what's positive, promoting feelings of contentment and peace before sleep. We will explore specific techniques for breathing, writing, and meditation in the following chapters.

Gentle movements, like some light stretches or restorative yoga poses, can help release physical tension accumulated in the body throughout the day. Focusing on bodily sensations during movement also serves as a form of moving meditation, bringing attention to the present and facilitating muscle relaxation.

The most important thing in building your nightly ritual is not the complexity of the chosen activities, but the consistency with which you practice them. It's the daily repetition that creates the conditioning and strengthens the association between these actions and impending sleep. Start with a simple ritual, perhaps 15 to 30 minutes, and be patient with yourself. It may take some time for the effects to become noticeable, but perseverance will bring results. View this time not as another task to be completed, but as a gift you give yourself, a sacred moment of self-care and preparation for nightly renewal.

By committing to this nightly ritual, you are not only shaping a practical routine but also cultivating a gesture of reconnection with yourself. In a society that values productivity so highly, dedicating conscious time to closing the day is an act of gentle resistance – a reminder that rest is not a luxury, but a biological and emotional necessity. By creating this transition space, you begin to re-educate not only your body but also your perception of sleep, transforming it from a neglected moment into a point of return to your own integrity.

The cumulative effect of these small practices is profound. Gradually, they begin to reconfigure the mental and emotional patterns that often hinder falling asleep. Nighttime anxiety, repetitive thoughts, and hyperstimulation are replaced by a growing sense of predictability, comfort, and serenity. Ritualization becomes a kind of silent language between you and your nervous system, a tacit agreement that, at that moment, everything can slow down. And, like any language learned with affection and consistency, it deepens over time, until the simple act of lighting a candle or touching a page of paper becomes an invitation to repose.

With this, the nightly ritual ceases to be just a set of practices and becomes a state of mind, an intimate territory where presence and pause are cultivated. And it is in this space, between turning off the lights and welcoming the darkness, that sleep flourishes more easily. The body learns to trust, the mind learns to yield, and the silence of the night finally becomes a home.

Chapter 12
Conscious Breathing

Within the arsenal of practices that make up an effective nightly ritual, few are as accessible, immediate, and profoundly transformative as conscious breathing. This act, which we perform automatically thousands of times a day, holds immense power to regulate our internal state, serving as a direct bridge between our agitated mind and a state of calm and relaxation. Learning to consciously manage the rhythm and depth of our breath is like discovering a master key capable of modulating our nervous system, alleviating anxiety, and preparing the physiological ground for sleep. In this chapter, we will explore some simple and effective breathing techniques that can be easily incorporated into your pre-sleep routine, offering practical and immediate tools to calm the mind, reduce heart rate, and facilitate the natural and healthy transition between wakefulness and deep rest.

The connection between breathing and emotional state is intuitive. We notice that in moments of stress or fear, our breathing tends to become short, rapid, and shallow, concentrated in the upper chest. Conversely, when we are relaxed and calm, breathing naturally becomes slower, deeper, and abdominal. This relationship, however, works both ways. Just as our emotions affect breathing, we can intentionally use breathing to influence our emotions and physiological state. By adopting breathing patterns associated with relaxation, we send signals to the brain that we are safe and that it's possible to "turn off" the fight-or-flight response (sympathetic nervous system) and activate the rest-and-digest response (parasympathetic nervous system).

Activating the parasympathetic nervous system is crucial for sleep. It promotes a decrease in heart rate, blood pressure, and muscle tension, in addition to reducing the production of stress hormones like cortisol. Essentially, conscious breathing helps us move out of the alert state and into a state conducive to relaxation and regeneration. It's a way of communicating to our body, through the most fundamental language it knows – the rhythm of life – that the danger has passed and it can allow itself to rest.

One of the best-known and most effective techniques for quickly inducing relaxation is the 4-7-8 breath. Popularized by Dr. Andrew Weil, it is based on ancient pranayama (breath control) practices from yoga. The technique is simple and can be practiced sitting or lying comfortably. Start by completely emptying your lungs, exhaling all the air through your mouth with a soft "whoosh" sound. Then, close your mouth and inhale silently through your nose, mentally counting to four. Hold your breath, counting to seven. Finally, exhale completely through your mouth, again with a soft "whoosh" sound, counting to eight. This complete cycle (inhale 4, hold 7, exhale 8) constitutes one repetition. It's recommended to start with four repetitions and, with practice, gradually increase if desired. The key lies in the ratio and the prolonged exhalation, which has a particularly calming effect on the nervous system. The mental counting also helps focus attention, diverting intrusive thoughts.

Another valuable technique is alternate nostril breathing, known in yoga as Nadi Shodhana. This practice aims to balance the brain hemispheres and calm the mind. Sit comfortably with your spine erect. Use your right thumb to gently close your right nostril and inhale slowly and deeply through your left nostril. Then, use your right ring finger to close the left nostril and exhale completely through the right nostril. Keep the left nostril closed and inhale through the right nostril. Close the right nostril with your thumb and exhale through the left nostril. This complete cycle (inhale left, exhale right, inhale right, exhale left) constitutes one round. Continue for several rounds, maintaining a smooth, slow, and effortless rhythm. Alternate nostril breathing promotes a state of balance and tranquility, excellent for reducing anxiety and preparing the mind for sleep.

Diaphragmatic breathing, or abdominal breathing, is perhaps the most fundamental and natural way to breathe, although many of us, due to chronic stress, adopt a shallower, chest-based pattern. Retraining the body to breathe deeply from the diaphragm (the large muscle located at the base of the lungs) is extremely beneficial for relaxation. Lie comfortably on your back, with knees bent or supported by a pillow. Place one hand gently on your abdomen and the other on your chest. Inhale slowly through your nose, directing the air to the lower part of your lungs, so that the hand on your abdomen rises, while the hand on your chest remains relatively still. Exhale slowly through your mouth or nose, feeling the abdomen gently fall. Focus on making the breath slow, deep, and regular. Imagine your abdomen is a balloon gently inflating on the inhale and deflating on the exhale. Practicing diaphragmatic breathing for 5 to 10 minutes before sleep helps better oxygenate the body, massages internal organs, and sends a powerful relaxation signal to the nervous system.

The beauty of these techniques lies in their simplicity and the fact that breathing is always with us, available at any moment as an anchor to the present and a tool for self-regulation. They require no special equipment and can be practiced discreetly anywhere, although they are particularly effective when incorporated into the nightly ritual, in the comfort of your sleep sanctuary.

When starting the practice, be kind to yourself. The mind may wander, and it might take some time until the calming effects become more evident. What matters is intention and persistence. Start with a few minutes and gradually increase as you feel comfortable. Observe the sensations in your body – the heart rate slowing, muscles relaxing, the mind quieting. Use breathing as a gentle guide to lead you from a state of agitation to a state of serenity.

By integrating conscious breathing into your nightly ritual, you establish a direct line between the external world, with its noises and demands, and the internal universe of silence and presence. This simple but profound gesture of turning to the breath is like opening a door within yourself, an invitation to withdrawal and listening to the body in its natural rhythm. As the practice becomes habitual, breathing ceases to be just a technical exercise and transforms into a constant shelter – a silent way to return to balance whenever the day's tension threatens to invade the night.

The consistency of this practice teaches more than techniques: it reveals a new way of inhabiting time and one's own body. By inhaling with attention and exhaling with surrender, you begin to perceive subtle nuances – how the body responds to relief, how thoughts become less insistent, how sleep approaches without being forced. It's a delicate dance between control and surrender, where you actively participate in the process of calming yourself while learning to trust the intelligence of your own organism. Over time, conscious breathing can extend beyond the nightly ritual and become an ally in other areas of life, as an intimate and always accessible resource for emotional self-regulation.

Ultimately, cultivating this breathable space within the night is a silent gift offered to the body and soul. It is in this slow, intentional rhythm that rest reveals itself not as interruption, but as a natural continuation of care. Breathing then becomes more than survival: it becomes a gesture of affection, a way of touching life lightly, preparing the fertile ground where sleep can land gently and remain.

Chapter 13
Muscle Relaxation

While conscious breathing acts as an exquisite tool for calming the mind and modulating the nervous system, often the tension preventing us from relaxing and falling asleep is deeply lodged in our physical body. Tense shoulders, a clenched jaw, a stiff back – the stress and worries of the day frequently manifest as muscle contractions, many of which we aren't even aware. This residual physical tension sends alert signals to the brain, perpetuating the cycle of agitation and hindering surrender to rest. Fortunately, just as we can use breath to calm the mind, we can use the body itself as a direct ally in the slowing-down process, through a technique known as progressive muscle relaxation. This simple and effective method teaches us to actively recognize and dissolve accumulated tensions, promoting a state of deep physical tranquility that positively resonates with the central nervous system and facilitates the arrival of sleep.

Progressive muscle relaxation is based on a simple physiological principle: after a period of intense contraction, a muscle tends to relax more deeply than before. The technique involves deliberately tensing specific muscle groups for a short period (usually 5 to 7 seconds) and then abruptly releasing that tension, paying attention to the sensation of relaxation that follows (for about 15 to 20 seconds). By systematically going through different muscle groups of the body, from head to toe or vice versa, we learn to contrast the sensation of tension with that of relaxation, increasing our body awareness and our ability to voluntarily release contractions. This process not only relaxes the muscles themselves but also sends calming signals to the nervous system, helping reduce sympathetic activity (fight or flight) and promote the parasympathetic response (rest and digest). The practice can be comfortably performed in bed, shortly before sleep, making it a powerful resource for those whose insomnia is linked to anxiety, physical restlessness, or simply difficulty "switching off" the body after a busy day.

Find a comfortable position, lying on your back, arms alongside your body, legs slightly apart. Close your eyes and begin with a few slow, deep breaths, like those learned in the previous chapter, to start the relaxation process. The sequence usually starts at the feet and moves up the body, but can be adapted to individual preference. The important thing is to be systematic and not skip muscle groups. Let's describe an ascending sequence as an example:

Start with the feet. Tense the muscles of your feet, curling your toes down or up, as if trying to grip something with them. Hold the tension for about 5 seconds, focusing on the feeling of tightness. Then, abruptly release the tension and feel your feet relax completely. Notice the difference between tension and relaxation. Remain in this feeling of release for 15 to 20 seconds, breathing gently.

Move up to the calves. Flex your feet towards your face, as if trying to touch your shins with your toes, or point your feet downwards, tensing the calf muscles. Hold the contraction, feel the tightness, and then release. Let your calves become heavy and relaxed, noticing the absence of tension.

Continue to the thighs. Tense the muscles in the front and back of your thighs, pressing your knees together or trying to forcefully straighten your legs. Feel the powerful tension in these large muscles, and then release completely. Allow your thighs to become soft and heavy on the bed.

Now, the buttocks. Tense your glutes, squeezing them firmly. Hold for a few seconds and release. Feel your pelvis relax and settle more deeply onto the supporting surface.

Move to the abdomen. Contract your abdominal muscles, as if bracing for a light impact, pulling your navel towards your spine or pushing your belly outwards. Hold the tension and then release completely, allowing your breath to flow freely in the abdominal region.

Move up to the chest. Inhale deeply and hold your breath for a moment, tensing the muscles of your chest and upper back. Then, exhale and release all tension. Feel your chest open and relax.

Arms and hands. Clench your hands into tight fists and contract your biceps and triceps, as if showing off your muscles or pushing something. Feel the tension in your fists, forearms, and arms. Release abruptly, opening your hands and letting your arms become heavy and loose beside your body.

Shoulders. Raise your shoulders towards your ears, as if trying to touch them. Hold this tension in your upper back and neck. Then, drop your shoulders down, feeling the weight and relief in the area.

Neck. Carefully, press your head slightly back against the pillow or gently tilt it to one side and then the other, feeling the tension in the side muscles (avoid sudden or painful movements). Relax completely, finding a neutral and comfortable position for your head.

Finally, the face. Tense your facial muscles: frown your forehead, squeeze your eyes shut, clench your jaw (careful not to hurt your teeth), and make a grimace. Hold the tension for a few seconds and then release everything. Relax your forehead, eyelids, cheeks, and especially your jaw, letting your lips part slightly. Feel your entire face become soft and relaxed.

After going through all the muscle groups, remain lying down for a few minutes, enjoying the overall sensation of deep relaxation pervading your entire body. Notice how the mind also tends to become calmer and quieter when the body is free from tension. Breathe gently and allow yourself to simply be, surrendering to the stillness and drowsiness that may arise.

Regular practice of progressive muscle relaxation not only helps induce sleep but also increases body awareness throughout the day. You'll start to notice more easily where you accumulate tension and can use brief relaxation techniques to release it before it becomes chronic. It's a way of using the body as an instrument of self-knowledge and self-care, recognizing the intimate connection between the physical state and the mental state.

By making the body a conscious ally in the process of falling asleep, progressive muscle relaxation reveals itself as more than a technique – it's a path of reconciliation with one's own physicality. Instead of trying to silence the mind solely through force of thought, this practice teaches us to listen to the body's signals, recognize the small accumulated tensions we often ignore, and gently release the invisible weight we carry. Each relaxed muscle is an invitation to rest, a clear message sent to the nervous system that there's no longer a need to resist, only to repose.

Over time, this practice also deepens our intimacy with our own limits and needs. It shows us that relaxation isn't a state that happens by chance, but something that can be cultivated with intention and presence. The more we refine our bodily perception, the more easily we can intervene before stress silently and persistently takes hold. We learn to identify a tense shoulder as a request for a pause, a clenched jaw as a warning of emotional overload. And by responding with care and attention, we create a new form of internal dialogue – more compassionate, more attuned to integral well-being.

In the end, relaxing the body transforms into a gesture of surrender that opens space for true regeneration. By lying down each night and mindfully scanning the muscles that supported the day, you free them from the invisible burden of continuous effort. And it is in this state of tranquil surrender that sleep approaches, not as an imposition, but as a natural consequence of care. The body relaxes, the mind silences, and rest settles in, full and deserved.

Chapter 14
Sounds and Silences

Our journey through practical tools to enhance sleep now leads us to explore a sense often underestimated in its influence on rest: hearing. The sound environment surrounding us, especially at night, can be both a significant obstacle and a powerful ally in the process of falling asleep and maintaining peaceful sleep. From the disruptive noises of urban life to the profound quietness that seems to invite withdrawal, sounds and silences shape our nocturnal experience in subtle and profound ways. This chapter delves into the power of sound – and its absence – as a tool to induce relaxation, mask disturbances, and even influence our brainwaves, guiding us towards states more conducive to sleep. Learning to consciously manage our auditory environment and discover which sound stimuli work best for our individual constitution is another essential step towards transforming our nights and waking up with more vitality.

For many, especially those living in cities or noisy environments, absolute silence might seem an unattainable luxury. Traffic noise, sirens, neighbors, or even internal house noises can create a sonic backdrop that keeps the nervous system in a state of alert, even subliminally. These intermittent or constant sounds can make falling asleep difficult, cause micro-arousals that fragment sleep (often without our awareness), and generally decrease the restorative quality of rest. Therefore, seeking strategies to create an effective sound barrier in the bedroom is a fundamental starting point. This might involve measures like installing soundproof windows, using heavy curtains that absorb sound, sealing gaps in doors and windows, or, more simply and accessibly, using good quality earplugs. Creating a cocoon of relative silence allows the nervous system to relax more deeply, feeling safe to surrender to sleep.

However, for some people, absolute silence can be disconcerting or even anxiety-provoking. In the absence of external stimuli, the mind might turn inward, amplifying ruminative thoughts or the perception of internal bodily noises, like heartbeat or tinnitus. In these cases, or when external noises are impossible to eliminate completely, introducing controlled, calming sounds can be extremely beneficial. This is where concepts like white noise and other continuous sounds come in.

White noise is a sound containing all audible frequencies at equal intensity. Think of the sound of an off-air television, a fan, or a distant waterfall. Its primary function in the context of sleep is sound masking. By creating a constant and neutral sonic background, white noise makes sudden and disruptive sounds (like a door slamming or a horn honking) less noticeable, as they blend into the background noise instead of standing out abruptly in the silence. This helps create a more stable and predictable auditory environment, which can be very comforting for the brain and facilitate both falling asleep and staying asleep. There are also variations like pink noise (with more intensity in lower frequencies, like constant rain) or brown noise (even deeper, like strong ocean waves), which some people find more pleasant and relaxing. Dedicated white noise generators, smartphone apps, or even a fan can be used for this purpose.

Nature sounds are another popular and effective category for inducing relaxation. Sounds like gentle rain, ocean waves breaking on the shore, the crackling of a fireplace, birds singing in a forest, or the murmur of a stream have a proven calming effect on the nervous system. These sounds evoke a sense of peace, security, and connection with the natural world, helping reduce stress levels and slow down the mind. The predictability and absence of complex verbal or emotional content in these sounds allow the mind to relax without actively engaging. Many high-quality recordings are available on streaming platforms or apps, allowing you to bring the serenity of nature into your bedroom.

Music can also be a powerful ally, but choosing the right type is crucial. Music with lyrics, complex rhythms, or abrupt dynamic variations can be stimulating rather than relaxing. Ideally, opt for slow instrumental music, such as soft classical piano pieces, ambient music, new age, or compositions specifically created for relaxation and meditation. Binaural music is an interesting category to explore. It uses headphones to send sounds with slightly different frequencies to each ear. The brain, trying to process this difference, generates a third perceived frequency internally, corresponding to the difference between the two. It is claimed that by choosing the correct frequencies, it's possible to induce the brain into brainwave states associated with relaxation (alpha waves, 8-13 Hz) or even the initial stages of sleep (theta waves, 4-7 Hz). Although scientific research is still developing, many people report significant benefits from using binaural beats to relax and fall asleep.

The key to using sound as a sleep tool is experimentation and personalization. What works wonderfully for one person might be irritating for another. Dedicate some time to explore different types of sounds – white noise, pink noise, nature sounds, ambient music, binaural beats – and observe how your body and mind react to each. Pay attention if the sound helps you relax, divert attention from anxious thoughts, or mask disruptive noises. Adjust the volume to a comfortable level, present enough to have an effect, but not so loud as to become intrusive. Also consider using timers so the sound turns off automatically after you fall asleep, if you prefer silence during deep sleep, or leave it playing softly throughout the night if it helps prevent awakenings.

By learning to consciously manage the sound environment of your bedroom, whether cultivating silence or introducing calming sounds, you add another layer of intentional care to your sleep preparation. You transform what could be a source of disturbance into an active ally in the relaxation process.

This intentional listening, when it becomes part of the nightly ritual, teaches us to attune our relationship with the space we sleep in. It's not just about eliminating noise, but about shaping a sound environment that welcomes the body and mind in their transition to repose. By recognizing the subtle effects that different soundscapes have on our internal state, we begin to use them as instruments of self-regulation – carefully choosing what surrounds us at the moment we most need safety and serenity. This auditory curation transforms the bedroom into a sensory refuge, where every present sound contributes to silencing what isn't seen, but felt.

Furthermore, the act of listening itself becomes a meditative practice. By surrendering to the constancy of light rain or the slow tempo of soft music, we allow the mind to settle on something external, predictable, and benign. This helps dissolve internal noises – racing thoughts, late-night worries – without needing to fight them directly. In this context, sound and silence become two sides of the same coin: a space where the day's content can settle more gently. Instead of trying to escape mental agitation, we learn to redirect it to a safe place, where the body can disarm itself and sleep can arise as a natural consequence.

In this balance between sound that lulls and silence that welcomes, we discover a new way to prepare for the night. There is no universal formula, but there is a certainty: when we intentionally surround ourselves with sounds that nourish and calm, we offer our mind the same care we offer our body with a comfortable mattress or soft lighting. Rest begins long before closing the eyes – it begins in listening. And by tuning the environment so it softly sings the song of repose, we give sleep permission to arrive and, with it, the peace that renews.

Chapter 15
Inducing Aromas

Our sensory exploration in search of restorative sleep now leads us to the subtle and evocative realm of aromas. Smell, one of our most primal senses and directly connected to brain areas responsible for emotions and memories, offers a fascinating and effective pathway to influence our state of mind and prepare the body for rest. The practice of aromatherapy, which uses essential oils extracted from plants, flowers, barks, and resins, is based on the ability of certain fragrances to promote relaxation, alleviate anxiety, and induce a sense of calm conducive to sleep. In this chapter, we will learn about some of the most celebrated aromas for their sleep-inducing properties, explore different ways to incorporate them into our nightly ritual, and understand a bit more about how this olfactory connection acts as a powerful bridge between our body, mind, and the desired state of peaceful repose.

The relationship between aromas and states of mind is not new. Since time immemorial, various cultures have used incense, aromatic herbs, and oils in religious rituals, healing practices, and to promote well-being. The secret to this influence lies in the anatomy of our olfactory system. Aromatic molecules, when inhaled, travel directly to the olfactory bulb, which is intrinsically linked to the limbic system – the emotional center of the brain, responsible for regulating mood, memory, behavior, and basic physiological functions. Unlike other senses, smell has this direct line to emotions, without first passing through the thalamus, which acts as a relay center for other sensory information. That's why a particular scent can instantly evoke a vivid memory or alter our mood almost immediately. By choosing aromas with known relaxing properties, we can use this direct pathway to calm the nervous system and signal to the body that it's safe to relax.

Among the most studied and recommended aromas for promoting sleep, lavender (Lavandula angustifolia) reigns supreme. Its floral and gentle scent is known for its calming, anxiolytic, and mild sedative properties. Studies suggest that linalool, one of its main components, interacts with neurotransmitters like GABA, which has an inhibitory effect on the central nervous system, helping reduce mental agitation and promote muscle relaxation. Lavender can help lower heart rate, blood pressure, and skin temperature, preparing the body to fall asleep faster and improving overall sleep quality.

Chamomile, especially Roman (Anthemis nobilis) or German (Matricaria chamomilla), is another classic ally for peaceful sleep. Known for its sweet, herbal aroma, chamomile is often consumed as a relaxing tea, but its essential oil also possesses significant calming properties. It's believed that apigenin, a compound found in chamomile, binds to receptors in the brain similarly to some anxiolytic medications, promoting drowsiness and reducing anxiety. Its gentle effect makes it an excellent option for those seeking mild relaxation before bed.

Sandalwood (Santalum album), with its woody, warm, and exotic aroma, has been valued for centuries in spiritual practices for its grounding and centering properties. In aromatherapy for sleep, sandalwood is appreciated for its ability to calm the mind, relieve nervous tension, and promote a sense of inner peace. Its effect is less sedative and more balancing, helping silence mental noise and create an internal space conducive to deep rest and meditation.

Ylang-ylang (Cananga odorata), extracted from a tropical flower, has an intensely sweet and floral aroma, known for its aphrodisiac properties, but also for its relaxing and antidepressant effects. It can help reduce blood pressure, heart rate, and stress levels, alleviating feelings of anger, panic, or anxiety. Its exotic and enveloping scent can transform the bedroom environment, promoting a sense of well-being and tranquility that facilitates surrender to sleep. Other oils like marjoram, bergamot, neroli, and vetiver are also frequently cited for their relaxing properties and can be explored.

There are several practical and safe ways to incorporate these aromas into your nightly ritual. One of the most popular is the use of essential oil diffusers. These devices disperse microparticles of oil into the air, filling the room with the chosen fragrance. Turning on the diffuser in the bedroom about 30 minutes before bed can create a relaxing atmosphere and signal the start of your ritual. It's important to choose a good quality diffuser and use only pure, 100% natural essential oils.

Another simple option is a pillow or room spray. You can buy ready-made sprays or make your own by diluting a few drops of the chosen essential oil in grain alcohol and distilled water in a spray bottle. Lightly spraying on the pillow, sheets, or in the bedroom air before sleep allows you to gently inhale the aroma throughout the night.

Adding a few drops of essential oil to a warm bath or foot soak is a luxurious way to combine the benefits of hydrotherapy with aromatherapy. The heat of the water helps volatilize the oils, intensifying the aromatic experience and promoting deep muscle and mental relaxation. Remember to dilute essential oils in a carrier oil (like coconut or almond oil) or bath salts before adding to water, to avoid skin irritation.

A light massage with diluted essential oils can also be extremely relaxing. Massaging feet, shoulders, neck, or temples with a carrier oil infused with lavender or chamomile before bed can help relieve muscle tension and calm the mind through the combined touch and aroma. Dilution is crucial for topical application; generally, a few drops of essential oil per tablespoon of carrier oil are sufficient.

It's crucial to emphasize the importance of using essential oils with caution and respect. They are concentrated and potent substances. Research the quality of oils, follow dilution recommendations, and avoid ingestion or direct application to the skin without proper dilution. People with pre-existing medical conditions, pregnant or nursing women, or young children should consult a healthcare professional or qualified aromatherapist before using essential oils.

Choosing the ideal aroma is a personal journey. Experiment with different oils, paying attention to your individual reactions and preferences. What is relaxing for one person may not be for another. Observe which aromas bring you a genuine sense of calm, security, and well-being. Once you find your aromatic allies, integrate them into your nightly ritual consistently.

This consistency in the presence of aromas creates, over time, an unconscious link between a particular scent and the act of resting. Just as a melody can evoke a feeling, or an image can trigger a memory, the aroma becomes a sensory signal that prepares the body to gradually switch off. With repeated use, the brain learns to associate certain smells with states of tranquility, slowing mental activity and promoting a smoother transition to sleep. It's a positive conditioning that works gently, almost like a whisper, preparing the internal environment for withdrawal.

The strength of aromas lies in their subtlety: they don't need to dominate the space, just inhabit it delicately. The difference between a scent that invites relaxation and one that disturbs often lies in the dosage, purity, and alignment with personal taste. Therefore, using aromatherapy requires listening and presence. It's by paying attention to the body's reactions – the deepening breath, the easing chest, the dissolving thought – that we find our guide-aromas. And when this connection is established, it becomes part of our nocturnal environment as naturally as a favorite pillow or the welcoming dimness of the room.

Incorporating these aromas into the sleep ritual is more than adding a fragrance: it's building a sensory stage where rest is invited to arrive. It's an intimate gesture of care, returning us to the simplicity of the senses as a path to restoring balance. And thus, amidst lavender, chamomile, or the warmth of sandalwood, the bedroom transforms into a sanctuary of quietude, where the body can release the day's weight and the mind, enveloped in aroma and silence, finally allows itself to fall asleep.

Chapter 16
The Power of Light

Our exploration of practical tools for cultivating restorative sleep now leads us to consider one of the most powerful and omnipresent environmental elements in our lives: light. From the first ray of sun announcing dawn to the artificial glow of screens accompanying us late into the night, light exerts a profound and constant influence on our internal biology, acting as the primary conductor of our biological clock, the so-called circadian rhythm. Understanding the power of light and learning to manage our exposure to it throughout the day and night is fundamental to regulating the production of essential hormones like melatonin and, consequently, promoting a healthy and balanced sleep-wake cycle. This chapter delves into the science behind this vital connection and offers practical strategies for creating "light hygiene" in our environment, transforming light from a potential disruptor into a powerful ally for our physical and emotional well-being.

The circadian rhythm is an approximately 24-hour cycle that regulates a wide range of physiological processes in our body, including sleep, wakefulness, body temperature, hormone release, and metabolism. This internal clock, located in a small brain region called the suprachiasmatic nucleus (SCN), is genetically determined but needs daily synchronization with the external environment to stay aligned. The primary environmental cue (or *zeitgeber*, as known scientifically) for the SCN is the natural cycle of light and darkness. Light, especially sunlight rich in the blue spectrum, captured by the eyes, sends direct signals to the SCN, informing it about the time of day and adjusting our internal clock.

During the day, exposure to natural light, particularly in the morning, is crucial for suppressing the production of melatonin, the hormone that induces sleepiness. This suppression helps us feel alert, awake, and energized. Morning sunlight acts as a "reset" for the biological clock, ensuring it's correctly synchronized with the 24-hour cycle. Lack of adequate natural light exposure during the day, common for people spending most of their time indoors with insufficient artificial lighting, can lead to a "weak" or desynchronized biological clock, resulting in daytime sleepiness, lack of energy, and difficulty sleeping at night. Therefore, actively seeking sunlight in the morning, whether through a walk, having coffee outdoors, or working near a well-lit window, is a fundamental practice of light hygiene.

As the day progresses and night approaches, the natural decrease in light intensity and the shift in light hue (becoming warmer, reddish) signal to the SCN that it's time to start preparing the body for rest. In response to darkness, the pineal gland begins to produce and release melatonin into the bloodstream. Melatonin doesn't "knock you out" like a sedative, but acts as a "gate opener" for sleep, decreasing alertness, reducing body temperature, and facilitating the transition to sleep. Melatonin production usually begins a few hours before our habitual bedtime, peaks in the middle of the night, and gradually decreases as morning approaches.

The great challenge of modern life lies in our excessive exposure to artificial light during the night. Bright lamps, televisions, computers, tablets, and smartphones emit light, especially in the blue spectrum, which the SCN interprets as daylight. This nighttime exposure to artificial light, even at low intensity, can significantly suppress or delay melatonin release, confusing our biological clock and making it difficult to fall asleep. Staying in brightly lit environments or using electronic devices late into the night sends the brain the message that it's still daytime, sabotaging the natural signals that should prepare us for sleep. This is one of the main factors contributing to the epidemic of sleep problems in current society.

Fortunately, practical strategies and resources are available to mitigate the negative effects of nighttime artificial light and create healthier light hygiene. The first step is to reduce the intensity of home lighting in the hours leading up to sleep. Use lamps with dimmer, warm-toned bulbs (yellow, amber, or red) instead of bright, white ceiling lights. Installing dimmers allows you to adjust light intensity as needed. Avoid using electronic screens as much as possible in the two to three hours before bed. If you must use them, activate night modes or blue light filters available on most devices, which reduce blue spectrum emission and give the screen a warmer hue. For additional protection, consider using blue-light-blocking glasses. These glasses, with orange or reddish lenses, filter the light frequencies most disruptive to melatonin production and can be worn in the final hours of the day, especially if exposure to screens or bright lights is unavoidable. They allow you to carry out your evening activities without compromising the natural signaling for sleep as much.

Another interesting tool is timer lamps or smart bulbs that can be programmed to gradually decrease intensity and change the light hue throughout the evening, simulating an artificial sunset and helping induce relaxation. Similarly, there are alarm clocks that simulate sunrise, gradually increasing light intensity in the morning to promote a gentler, more natural awakening, instead of the jolt caused by an audible alarm.

Creating "light hygiene" therefore involves consciously managing our light exposure over 24 hours: maximizing bright natural light during the day, especially in the morning, and minimizing bright artificial light, especially blue light, during the night. It's about aligning our luminous environment with our natural biological rhythm, respecting the signals our bodies have evolved to recognize over millennia. By implementing these strategies, we use the power of light not as an obstacle, but as a powerful tool to regulate our sleep, mood, and energy levels. Small changes in how we interact with light can have a significant impact on the quality of our rest and, by extension, our overall physical and emotional health. It's an invitation to observe our environment with new eyes, recognizing the subtle but constant influence of lighting on our well-being, and to take practical steps to create a home that supports, rather than disturbs, our natural cycle of activity and repose.

Beyond its practical applications, the relationship between light and circadian rhythm invites us to a deeper reconnection with the natural cycles governing life. We live in an era where the artificial has imposed itself on the natural, and we often forget that our bodies still respond to signals as primal as sunrise and sunset. Light, in this context, ceases to be just a technical element to regulate and becomes a language our body intuitively understands—a language that, if used well, can re-establish an interrupted dialogue between modern humans and the nature that shaped them. Returning to this harmony is, simultaneously, an act of self-care and a reclaiming of what is essential.

This alignment with light cycles can also become a mindfulness practice. Observing how light changes throughout the day, adjusting activities according to this dance of shadows and brightness, noticing how the body responds to each luminous nuance—all this brings us closer to a more present, more conscious lifestyle. Instead of fighting against the biological clock, we learn to collaborate with it, respecting its times and needs. Thus, light hygiene transcends mere technique and transforms into a broader attitude of respect for our own rhythm, promoting not only more restorative sleep but also a more harmonious experience of time and ourselves. By understanding light as a silent and potent ally, we open space for subtle yet lasting transformations in our quality of life. Cultivating this attentive gaze towards our surroundings, recognizing the impact it has on our organism, and consciously adjusting these stimuli becomes one of the most accessible and effective ways to recover the serenity of nights and the vigor of days. Light, after all, can be much more than clarity: it can be the invisible thread intertwining health, balance, and presence in every moment of our daily lives.

Chapter 17
Temperature and Texture

Continuing our investigation into shaping the environment to favor sleep, we now turn our attention to two sensory elements of great impact, though sometimes overlooked: temperature and texture. Just like light and sound, the thermal sensation of our body and environment, as well as the touch of materials surrounding us during the night, play a crucial role in our ability to relax, fall asleep, and maintain deep, uninterrupted sleep. Our body has intricate thermoregulatory mechanisms closely linked to the sleep-wake cycle, and the tactile comfort provided by appropriate bedding and clothing can make the difference between a night of restlessness and truly cozy rest. This chapter explores the science behind the relationship between temperature, texture, and sleep, offering practical guidance to optimize these aspects and create a cocoon of absolute sensory comfort, where every physical detail conspires in favor of mental disengagement and deepening repose.

Body temperature follows a natural circadian rhythm, peaking in the late afternoon or early evening and progressively decreasing as we prepare for sleep. This drop in core temperature is an important biological signal that facilitates sleep onset. For this drop to occur efficiently, the temperature of our surrounding environment needs to be slightly lower. An excessively hot room hinders body heat dissipation, making it harder to fall asleep and potentially leading to more restless sleep with more awakenings. Conversely, a room that's too cold can also be uncomfortable and require the body to expend energy to stay warm, which also interferes with sleep.

Although thermal sensitivity varies from person to person, most research suggests that the ideal ambient temperature for sleeping falls within a relatively cool range, generally between 18 and 21 degrees Celsius (64 to 70 degrees Fahrenheit). Keeping the room within this range helps the body reach and maintain the slightly lower core temperature needed for quality sleep. This can be achieved through air conditioning, fans, or simply opening windows to let in fresh air before bed (if external conditions allow and are safe). It's important to note that the ideal temperature is one where you feel comfortable without needing excessive blankets or, conversely, without feeling hot or sweating. Observing your own sensitivity and making gradual adjustments is key.

In addition to ambient temperature, the choice of sleepwear and bedding directly influences our thermoregulation during the night. Opting for pajamas or nightgowns made of natural, breathable fabrics like cotton, linen, silk, or bamboo allows air to circulate and moisture (sweat) to be absorbed and evaporated, helping keep the skin dry and body temperature more stable.

Synthetic fabrics like polyester or nylon tend to trap heat and moisture, potentially leading to overheating and discomfort. The amount of clothing also matters; dress appropriately for the room temperature, avoiding excess layers that might cause heat. For some, sleeping nude (or with minimal clothing) can facilitate the body's natural thermoregulation.

Bedding – sheets, blankets, duvets, and pillows – also deserves special attention. As with sleepwear, prefer natural and breathable materials for sheets, such as good quality cotton (percale or sateen), linen, or bamboo. The choice of blanket or duvet should consider the season and your personal sensitivity to cold. Ideally, have options that allow layering as needed, rather than a single very heavy duvet that might cause overheating on milder nights. Some people also benefit from using weighted blankets, which apply gentle, constant pressure on the body, promoting a sense of security and relaxation similar to a hug, potentially calming the nervous system and improving sleep quality, especially for those suffering from anxiety or restless legs syndrome.

The mattress and pillow are key pieces for physical comfort and, indirectly, thermal regulation. Mattresses made with materials that retain heat, like certain dense memory foams, can contribute to nighttime overheating. Seeking mattresses with technologies promoting air circulation or using more breathable materials, like natural latex or pocket springs with comfort layers of natural fibers, can make a difference. Similarly, pillows made of synthetic materials can retain heat around the head and neck. Options with natural fillings (like feathers, down, or latex) or cooling technologies may offer greater thermal comfort. Above all, the mattress and pillow must provide adequate support for your spine and preferred sleeping position, avoiding pain and discomfort that fragment sleep. Good support and tactile comfort are non-negotiable for restorative rest.

Seasonal changes obviously require adjustments. In summer, besides adjusting room temperature, taking a lukewarm bath (not cold, as cold can initially constrict blood vessels and hinder heat loss) before bed, using lighter bedding, and ensuring good ventilation can be helpful. In winter, the challenge is to keep the room comfortably warm without excessively drying the air (which can irritate airways). Using layers of bedding, warm socks (as cold feet can hinder falling asleep), and, if necessary, a heater with a thermostat can help. A humidifier might be useful if the air becomes too dry due to heating.

The key to optimizing temperature and texture for your sleep is self-observation and personalization. Pay attention to your body's signals. Do you wake up sweating or feeling cold? Does your mattress or pillow cause discomfort? Do your sheets feel rough or too warm? Make small adjustments and observe the impact on your sleep quality. Experiment with different fabrics, levels of covering, or room temperatures until you find the combination that provides maximum sensory comfort. Creating an environment that pleases your thermal and tactile senses is fundamental to promoting the deep relaxation necessary for sleep. When we feel physically comfortable, safe, and embraced by the materials surrounding us and the ambient temperature, we send our brain the message that everything is okay, that we can let down our guard and surrender to rest. Every physical detail – the softness of the sheet, the weight of the blanket, the coolness of the air – contributes to this state of mental disengagement and deepening sleep.

Beyond immediate comfort, attention to temperature and texture represents an act of listening to the body—a subtle gesture of intimacy with oneself. By tuning our perception to these stimuli, we learn to recognize the nuances of our nocturnal well-being and respond to them with careful choices. Sleep, after all, is not just about closing the eyes, but about allowing the body and mind to find common ground for repose. By adjusting the environment to our sensory needs, we create a kind of silent ritual, in which each physical element transforms into an invitation to release the day's tensions.

This sensitivity to touch and temperature also reconnects us with the importance of self-care in the daily routine. By prioritizing fabrics that gently embrace the skin, thermal sensations that favor relaxation, and choosing materials that respect our physiological individuality, we cultivate not only an environment conducive to rest but also a more attentive and compassionate relationship with our own limits. Sleeping well, in these terms, ceases to be an accidental privilege and becomes a conscious project of personal care, a construction that begins in the details and reflects broadly in our disposition, mood, and mental clarity.

Thus, by transforming the bed into a sensory refuge precisely adjusted to our needs, we revalue sleep as a complete experience—not just biological, but emotional and affective. We create, night after night, a space that welcomes us as we are, respecting the body's rhythm and the desire for pause. And it is in this gesture of delicacy towards our own senses that sleep gains depth, truly restores, and becomes a renewed source of balance and vitality.

Chapter 18
Nutrition and Sleep

Our exploration of tools to cultivate restorative sleep would not be complete without addressing a fundamental aspect of our daily routine: nutrition. What we choose to eat and drink, especially in the hours leading up to rest, exerts a direct and significant influence on our brain chemistry, hormone levels, and overall ability to relax and fall asleep peacefully. The relationship between nutrition and sleep is bidirectional – what we eat affects how we sleep, and how we sleep affects our food choices the next day. Understanding this intrinsic connection and learning to make conscious nutritional choices, particularly in the evening, is another essential step in building a solid foundation for restorative nights. This chapter delves into this relationship, highlighting foods and nutrients that can favor sleep, warning about substances that impair it, and offering guidance on meal timing and healthy nighttime snack options, showing that what we put on our plate at night can be a powerful ally or a silent saboteur of our rest.

The human body needs certain nutrients to produce neurotransmitters and hormones essential for sleep regulation. Serotonin, a neurotransmitter associated with well-being and relaxation, is a precursor to melatonin, the key hormone that induces sleepiness. To produce serotonin, the body needs an amino acid called tryptophan, which we don't produce naturally and must obtain through diet. Foods rich in tryptophan include turkey, chicken, eggs, fish, dairy products, nuts, seeds (like pumpkin and sesame), and legumes (like chickpeas and lentils). Consuming these foods throughout the day, and perhaps a small portion of complex carbohydrates at night (which help tryptophan cross the blood-brain barrier), can support the natural production of serotonin and, consequently, melatonin.

Some foods contain melatonin directly or substances that aid its production. Bananas, for example, are rich in potassium and magnesium, which help relax muscles, and also contain tryptophan. Oats are another excellent source of melatonin and complex carbohydrates that promote a gradual release of energy. Nuts, especially almonds and Brazil nuts, offer magnesium and melatonin. Cherries, particularly tart varieties, are one of the few natural food sources of melatonin and have been linked in studies to improved sleep duration and quality. Including these foods in the diet, especially as part of a light nighttime snack, can be beneficial.

Calming teas, such as chamomile, lemon balm, valerian, or passionflower, are traditional remedies for insomnia and relaxation. As we saw, chamomile contains apigenin, with anxiolytic effects. Valerian seems to interact with GABA receptors in the brain, promoting a mild sedative effect (although it should be used with caution and guidance, as it can cause daytime drowsiness in some people). Drinking a warm, caffeine-free cup of tea as part of the nightly ritual can be a comforting and effective way to signal to the body that it's time to slow down.

On the other hand, certain substances and eating habits can seriously impair sleep. Caffeine is perhaps the best known. Present in coffee, black tea, green tea, mate tea, chocolate, cola-based sodas, and some medications, caffeine is a powerful stimulant that blocks adenosine receptors in the brain – the substance that accumulates throughout the day and makes us feel sleepy. Caffeine can remain in the body for many hours (its half-life is about 5 to 6 hours), meaning a cup of coffee in the mid-afternoon can still affect your ability to fall asleep at night. It's recommended to avoid caffeine for at least 6 to 8 hours before bedtime.

Alcohol, although it may initially cause drowsiness and help you fall asleep faster, has a highly disruptive effect on sleep architecture later in the night. It suppresses REM sleep, essential for memory consolidation and emotional processing, and can lead to frequent awakenings in the second half of the night, resulting in fragmented and non-restorative sleep. Furthermore, alcohol relaxes throat muscles, which can worsen snoring and sleep apnea. Limiting or avoiding alcohol consumption, especially near bedtime, is crucial for sleep quality.

Heavy, fatty, fried, or very spicy meals require significant effort from the digestive system and can cause discomfort, heartburn, indigestion, or reflux, making it difficult to relax and fall asleep. The body needs to divert energy to digestion, which can slightly raise body temperature and interfere with sleepiness signals. Ideally, have the last main meal of the day at least two to three hours before going to bed, allowing sufficient time for initial digestion.

Excessive refined sugar and simple carbohydrates at night can also be problematic. They cause rapid spikes in blood glucose, followed by sharp drops, which can lead to nighttime awakenings when sugar levels fall too low. Additionally, a high-sugar diet can promote inflammation and negatively affect hormone production related to sleep. Opting for complex carbohydrates (like whole grains, legumes, and vegetables) and lean proteins in the evening meal promotes a more stable energy release.

If hunger strikes before bed, the strategy is to opt for a light, small snack that combines some complex carbohydrates with a source of tryptophan or magnesium. Some suggestions include: a small banana with a handful of almonds; half a cup of plain yogurt with some nuts; a slice of whole-wheat bread with peanut butter (sugar-free); or a glass of warm milk (which contains tryptophan and evokes childhood associations of comfort). Avoid large, sugary, or fatty snacks.

In summary, nutrition offers a tangible and tasty path to positively influence our sleep. It's not about following restrictive diets, but about making conscious choices, especially at the end of the day. Prioritize whole, nutritious foods, include sources of tryptophan and magnesium, avoid stimulants like caffeine and alcohol at night, have your last main meal well in advance, and opt for light, healthy nighttime snacks if needed. Paying attention to what and when we eat is another way to honor our body and create the ideal conditions for it to perform its essential nightly work of repair and renewal.

Far beyond the simple act of eating, the way we choose to nourish our bodies at night reveals a deeper commitment to care and balance. When we understand that certain foods can act as natural catalysts for rest and that our habits at the table directly impact sleep quality, we begin to see evening meals as an intentional gesture of preparation for repose. This shift in perspective transforms dinner and pre-sleep snacks into rituals of slowing down, where each dietary choice contributes to a physiological and emotional process of gradually disengaging from the day. Instead of viewing food merely as fuel, we start perceiving it as part of a sensitive mechanism that harmonizes body and mind in the crossing to night.

In this context, nutritional care also becomes an opportunity for reconnection with one's own rhythm. We often live at an accelerated pace, eating hastily, at irregular times, and without attention to what we are actually ingesting. By bringing awareness to the effects of food on sleep, we rediscover the importance of listening to our internal signals and respecting the cycles that sustain us. A light, nutritious, and comforting meal at the end of the day can be more than healthy: it can be soothing, almost therapeutic. And it is precisely in this everyday detail—a simple dish, warm tea, a choice made with attention—that lies one of the most accessible and effective paths to transforming turbulent nights into restorative rests.

By integrating nutrition and sleep as interdependent dimensions of well-being, we broaden our view of what it means to truly rest. Sleeping well is not an isolated event, but the result of small conscious decisions that accumulate throughout the day and, especially, in the hours preceding it. When we eat with respect for our bodies, we make space for them to reciprocate with calmer nights and more energetic days. And so, with simple yet intentional food choices, we reaffirm daily the idea that caring for sleep is, in essence, caring for life.

Chapter 19
Visualization Techniques

As we advance in our repertoire of practical tools to cultivate sleep, we arrive at a technique involving the creative power of our own mind: visualization. Often, the biggest obstacle to falling asleep isn't physical tension or environmental discomfort, but incessant mental activity – the whirlwind of thoughts, worries, plans, and memories that seem to take on a life of their own when we lay our head on the pillow. Creative visualization offers a gentle and effective path to calm this agitation, directing the mind's focus away from anxious ruminations and guiding it towards more serene states conducive to rest. It involves using our innate ability to imagine as a portal to deep relaxation, transforming the mind, often perceived as an adversary to sleep, into a powerful ally in the process of slowing down and peacefully falling asleep.

Visualization works because the human brain doesn't always clearly distinguish between a lived experience and a vividly imagined one. When we visualize a calm and safe scenario, we activate the same neural networks that would be activated if we were actually in that place. This, in turn, influences our autonomic nervous system, helping decrease the stress response (sympathetic) and activate the relaxation response (parasympathetic). Guided imagery can, therefore, induce real physiological changes, such as decreased heart rate, blood pressure, and muscle tension, creating an internal state favorable to sleep. Furthermore, by offering the mind a pleasant and absorbing focus, visualization helps interrupt the cycle of repetitive and anxious thoughts that frequently keep us awake.

There are numerous ways to practice visualization for sleep, and the key is to find or create scenarios that personally resonate with you, evoking feelings of peace, safety, and comfort. The practice usually begins by finding a comfortable position in bed, closing your eyes, and starting with a few slow, deep breaths to begin relaxing the body and mind. Then, you can start building the chosen mental image, involving as many senses as possible to make it more real and engaging.

A common approach is visualizing tranquil natural settings. Imagine yourself in a place you find deeply relaxing: perhaps a deserted beach at sunset, with the gentle sound of waves, the warm breeze on your skin, and the warm colors of the sky. Feel the soft sand beneath your feet, hear the distant cry of seagulls, smell the salty sea air. Allow yourself to walk slowly along the beach, feeling the tension leave your body with each step, or simply lie on the sand and feel the sun gently warming your skin. Other options might be a silent forest, with sunlight filtering through tall trees, the smell of damp earth, and the sound of a nearby stream; or a flowery meadow on a spring day, with the soft buzz of bees and the fragrance of flowers. The important thing is to choose a setting that brings you an immediate sense of calm and security. Explore the sensory details: the colors, sounds, smells, textures, temperature. The more vivid and detailed the image, the more absorbing it will become for the mind.

Another technique involves imaginary journeys. You might visualize yourself gently floating on a soft cloud, feeling light and weightless, watching the landscape pass peacefully below. Or perhaps imagine slowly descending a spiral staircase, where each step represents a deeper level of relaxation, feeling your body become heavier and your mind calmer with each downward step. It could be a boat trip down a calm river, gliding smoothly through the water under a starry sky. These symbolic journeys help create a sense of detachment from the day's worries and induce a state of progressive relaxation.

Encounters with comforting figures can also be used. Imagine being welcomed by a loving and protective presence – it could be a spiritual figure, a loved one (real or imaginary), or simply a warm, golden light enveloping you in safety and peace. Feel the warmth, love, and acceptance emanating from this presence, allowing all your tensions and fears to dissolve. This approach can be particularly helpful for those dealing with feelings of loneliness or anxiety at bedtime.

Beyond these examples, you are encouraged to create your own personalized visualization. Think of places, real or imaginary, that convey the feelings of peace, safety, comfort, and happiness you wish to cultivate before sleep. It could be a happy childhood memory, the feeling of being in your ideal home, or a completely fantastical scenario. The important thing is that the image is positive, relaxing, and meaningful to you. Don't worry about "getting it right"; the goal isn't to create a mental masterpiece, but to engage the imagination in a way that calms the nervous system.

During practice, it's normal for the mind to wander or for intrusive thoughts to arise. When this happens, simply acknowledge the thought without judgment and gently redirect your attention back to the visualization. Be patient and persistent. Like any skill, visualization becomes easier and more effective with regular practice. Incorporate it into your nightly ritual, dedicating 10 to 20 minutes to this inner journey.

Creative visualization is a powerful tool because it reminds us of our mind's intrinsic ability to shape our internal experience. Instead of being passive victims of our racing thoughts, we can actively choose to direct our imagination to create states of serenity and well-being. By making the mind an ally in the process of slowing down, we not only facilitate the arrival of sleep but also cultivate greater emotional resilience and a deeper connection with our own inner creative power.

Such practice not only aids the transition to sleep but also offers an intimate space for self-care and emotional self-regulation. By consciously choosing scenarios that evoke well-being, the practitioner strengthens brain circuits associated with safety, tranquility, and satisfaction, creating an internal repertoire accessible even during more difficult waking moments. Over time, these images become internal resources, almost like psychic refuges allowing access to a sense of peace even on turbulent days. The repetition of these imaginative states transforms visualization into a solid bridge between daily stress and the quietude of rest.

Furthermore, visualization offers a delicate alternative to forced attempts at falling asleep, which often only reinforce frustration and insomnia. Instead of fighting wakefulness, the practitioner engages in a pleasant experience, which in itself changes the relationship with bedtime. This reframes lying down as an opportunity for quiet pleasure, not a battlefield against fatigue or a restless mind. This shift in perspective is subtle but transformative: sleeping ceases to be a goal to be conquered and becomes a natural consequence of a serene dive into the inner world.

With practice and intention, visualization reveals itself as an art of inhabiting one's own imagination with kindness and presence. More than a technique for sleeping, it becomes a way of cultivating loving inner listening, welcoming one's emotions, and redirecting attention to states favoring repose. By allowing the mind to create images of calm and beauty, we take a firm step towards quieter nights and, by extension, a fuller, more integrated experience of our own rhythms and needs.

Chapter 20
Nightly Writing

After exploring techniques that calm the body through breathing, muscle relaxation, and managing the sensory environment, and that direct the mind through visualization, we now turn our attention to an introspective and profoundly liberating tool: writing. The act of putting thoughts, feelings, and worries on paper before sleep can function as a powerful practice of mental and emotional cleansing, a means of emptying the mind of the day's accumulation and creating an internal space of greater clarity and tranquility to welcome sleep. Nightly writing, whether structured or free-form, offers a safe and silent channel to externalize what troubles us, organize ideas, celebrate small victories, or simply record the passage of time, transforming into an intimate instrument of reconnection with the inner self and reduction of the mental noise that so often prevents us from falling asleep peacefully.

Often, the difficulty in falling asleep lies in taking unresolved worries, unfinished conversations, pending tasks, or unprocessed emotions from the day to bed. The mind continues to spin around these issues, like a scratched record, preventing the relaxation necessary for sleep. Therapeutic writing acts as an escape valve. By transferring these mental contents to paper, we create a healthy distance from them. They cease to be just an internal whirlwind and become something concrete, external to us, that can be observed, understood, and, in a sense, released, at least for that night. It's like unloading a heavy backpack before lying down; the relief can be immediate and significant.

There are several approaches to nightly writing, and you can experiment and adapt those that resonate most with your personality and current needs. One of the simplest and most effective forms is journaling or free writing. Reserve a few minutes before starting your relaxation ritual to sit with a notebook and pen (prefer paper over screen, to avoid blue light and the temptation of digital distractions) and simply write whatever comes to mind. Don't worry about grammar, style, or coherence. Allow yourself to vent about the day's challenges, express frustrations, fears, or joys. Write about what's worrying you, detailing the situation and your feelings about it. Often, the simple act of naming and describing a concern reduces its intensity. You can ask yourself questions on paper: "What really bothers me about this situation? What's the worst possible scenario? What can I do about it tomorrow?" This exploratory writing helps clarify emotions and gain perspective.

A powerful variation is gratitude writing. As briefly mentioned in the chapter on rituals, dedicating a few minutes to list three to five things you felt grateful for that day – however small – has a profound effect on our emotional state. It shifts the mind's focus from what's lacking or went wrong to what we have and what brought us joy, contentment, or comfort. It could be a stranger's smile, a successfully completed task, a moment of connection with a loved one, the taste of a meal, or the beauty of a sunset. Cultivating gratitude through writing before sleep helps end the day on a positive note, promoting feelings of peace and satisfaction highly conducive to sleep.

For those whose minds race with planning and to-do lists, writing can be used pragmatically to calm this anxiety. Take a moment to jot down all the tasks, ideas, or reminders swirling in your head for the next day. Create an organized list or a brief action plan. By putting this information on paper, you signal to your mind that it's safe, recorded, and can be revisited in the morning. This frees the brain from the need to mentally rehearse these pending items during the night, allowing it to relax more easily. It's like telling your mind: "It's all written down, now we can rest."

Writing can also be used as a space for conscious venting. If you're dealing with intense emotions like anger, sadness, or resentment, writing about them rawly and honestly, without censorship, can be extremely cathartic. Allow yourself to express everything you're feeling on paper, knowing it's a safe and private space. You could even write a letter (which doesn't need to be sent) to someone you have a conflict with, expressing your feelings. The goal isn't to find immediate solutions, but to release emotional intensity, preventing it from accumulating and disturbing your sleep. After writing, you can symbolically tear up or keep the paper, whichever feels more liberating.

Besides clearing the mind before sleep, writing can be a valuable tool for tracking your sleep and dream patterns, as suggested in the chapter on personal diagnosis and which will be further detailed later with the sleep diary. Keeping a notebook beside the bed to briefly note how the night's sleep went, the time you woke up, how you felt, and any dreams you remember can provide valuable insights into your patterns and the impact of the practices you are implementing. Recording dreams, even fragmented ones, can also be a fascinating way to dialogue with your unconscious.

To start your nightly writing practice, you can use some prompts or reflective questions if free writing seems daunting at first: What was most challenging today? What did I learn? What am I grateful for? What brought me joy? What do I need to release before sleep? What are my intentions for tomorrow? How do I feel right now? Choose one or two questions that resonate with you or create your own. The important thing is to find a writing routine that works for you, without it becoming another stressful obligation. Five to ten minutes can be sufficient. Use a notebook dedicated to this practice, making it a special object in your ritual.

By adopting writing as an ally for sleep, you create not only a channel for emotional expression but also a space for listening and inner care. Unlike the disordered mental dialogue that often dominates the moments before sleep, writing imposes a slower, more deliberate rhythm that invites presence and observation.

This movement of making visible what was previously just sensation or scattered thought acts as a form of containment, a symbolic frame allowing the mind to feel safer and less overwhelmed. There's something profoundly therapeutic in the simple gesture of putting words on paper – it's like building a bridge between internal chaos and external serenity, a passage gently leading to repose.

This practice also subtly strengthens emotional autonomy. By writing, you position yourself as an active subject facing your own experiences: you name, interpret, choose what to keep and what to let go. Over time, this habit can expand beyond the nighttime moment, influencing how you perceive and handle the day's events. And even if the immediate goal is sleep, the benefits extend to mental clarity, anxiety reduction, and cultivating a sense of inner coherence. Writing, when done with authenticity and openness, ceases to be just a technique and becomes almost a gesture of welcoming – a kind of silent hug we give ourselves at the end of each journey.

Incorporating writing into the nightly ritual is, therefore, much more than filling pages: it's creating a sacred interval between the world's noise and the silence necessary for sleep. In this intimate space, where everything can be said without rush or judgment, the mind finds permission to rest and the body, safety to surrender to sleep. And it is thus, between loose words, sincere questions, and written silences, that many restless nights begin to transform into nights of peace.

Chapter 21
Nightly Meditation

Concluding our exploration of practical tools to enhance sleep, we arrive at one of the most profound and transformative practices for cultivating inner calm and preparing the mind for rest: meditation. Often associated with images of monks in remote mountains, meditation, in its essence, is training in attention and awareness, a skill accessible to everyone that can be adapted simply and effectively for bedtime. Nightly meditation does not seek to empty the mind – an often frustrating goal – but rather to learn to observe thoughts and sensations without identifying with them, to anchor attention in the present moment, and to cultivate a state of serenity that naturally invites sleep. By practicing meditation before sleep, we not only facilitate the transition to rest but also develop greater resilience to stress and a deeper connection with ourselves.

The benefits of meditation for sleep are well-documented. Regular practice helps reduce levels of cortisol, the stress hormone, which, as we saw, is a major enemy of sleep when elevated at night. Meditation activates the parasympathetic nervous system, promoting a decrease in heart rate, blood pressure, and muscle tension, creating a physiological state conducive to relaxation. On a mental level, it teaches us to recognize repetitive and anxious thought patterns without getting carried away by them. By observing thoughts passing like clouds in the sky, instead of engaging with each one, we gradually reduce mental noise and create space for stillness. Meditation cultivates presence – the ability to be fully in the here and now – which, in itself, is a powerful antidote to worries about the past or future that so often keep us awake.

There are several meditation techniques that can be adapted for the nightly ritual. It's not necessary to sit in uncomfortable positions; many of these practices can be performed comfortably lying in bed. The important thing is to find an approach that resonates with you and practice it consistently.

Mindfulness meditation is an excellent starting point. It involves directing attention, intentionally and without judgment, to the experience of the present moment. A simple way to practice in bed is to focus on the breath. Observe the sensation of air entering and leaving the nostrils, or the gentle movement of the abdomen rising and falling with each respiratory cycle. Don't try to control the breath, just observe it as it is. When the mind wanders (which is perfectly normal), acknowledge where it went – a thought, a worry, a sound – and gently bring the attention back to the breath. Each time you do this, you are strengthening your mindfulness "muscle." Practice for 5, 10, or 15 minutes, using the breath as your constant anchor to the present.

The body scan is another mindfulness technique particularly effective for relaxing the body and inducing sleep. Lying comfortably, direct your attention sequentially to different parts of the body, starting from the toes and slowly moving up to the top of the head. For each part (feet, ankles, calves, knees, thighs, etc.), simply observe the sensations present – warmth, cold, tingling, weight, tension, or perhaps no particular sensation. Don't try to change anything, just observe with curiosity and acceptance. If you find areas of tension, you can imagine breathing into that area, and as you exhale, release the tension. The body scan helps reconnect the mind with the body, release unconscious tensions, and induce a state of deep relaxation, often leading to sleep even before completing the exercise.

Guided meditation can be a great option for beginners or for those days when the mind is particularly restless. Numerous recordings are available (on apps, websites, or streaming platforms) with narrations guiding the listener through relaxing visualizations (like those described in Chapter 19), mindfulness practices, or positive affirmations focused on sleep and relaxation. The calm voice of the guide serves as an external focus that helps maintain attention and direct the mind towards a quieter state. Look for meditations specifically created for sleep, which usually end in silence or with soft music, allowing you to fall asleep naturally.

Observing thoughts is a slightly more advanced but very powerful practice. Instead of fighting thoughts or trying to silence them, you adopt the stance of a neutral observer. Imagine your thoughts are clouds passing in the sky, cars passing on a road, or leaves floating down a river. Acknowledge each thought that arises, label it briefly (e.g., "thought about work," "worry," "memory"), and let it go, without clinging to it or judging it. Observe the space between thoughts. This practice helps disidentify from the mental stream, realizing you are not your thoughts, and reducing the power they have over your emotional state. Over time, the mind tends to calm down naturally.

To build a nightly meditative ritual adapted to your reality, start small. Five minutes of consistent meditation is more beneficial than an sporadic hour. Choose the technique you like best and establish a regular time, preferably as part of your wind-down ritual before sleep. Create a conducive environment, with low light and silence (or use relaxing sounds, if you prefer). Adopt a comfortable posture, whether sitting or lying down. Remember that the goal is not to achieve a special state or stop thinking, but to cultivate presence, acceptance, and kindness towards yourself. Some days meditation will feel easy and relaxing, other days the mind will be more restless. Welcome all experiences as part of the process.

Transforming meditation into an accessible and enjoyable habit is a valuable investment not only for the quality of your sleep but for your quality of life as a whole. It teaches us to navigate internal turbulence with more equanimity, reduce reactivity to stress, and cultivate a sense of inner peace independent of external circumstances. This practice, when cultivated regularly, becomes a true inner safe harbor, accessible at any time, including on nights when sleep seems most distant.

By establishing a space of quietude before sleep, you gradually re-educate the body and mind to associate this moment with rest, not with worry or agitation. Even if restlessness persists on some days, the simple decision to sit or lie down with intention and attention already signals a gesture of self-care—a gentle reminder that rest begins within, not without.

Beyond the immediate effects on sleep, the fruits of nightly meditation subtly extend into the following day. The mind awakens clearer, mood tends to be more stable, and daily challenges, though they remain, seem less oppressive. This happens because, by training the mind at night to return to the present gently, we create more skillful mental pathways for dealing with emotions and thoughts, even outside the formal practice time. Repetition, in this sense, is an ally: the more familiar we become with this state of presence, the more natural it becomes in all contexts.

Thus, allowing yourself this silent encounter before sleep is more than a technique—it's a gesture of reconnection. By creating this internal space for listening and welcoming, we gradually dissolve the layers of tension accumulated during the day and clear the path for a sleep born of care, not exhaustion. And it is in this care that the true restorative power of the night resides.

Chapter 22
Falling Asleep with Awareness

After exploring the fundamentals of sleep and delving into a wide range of practical techniques – from creating a physical sanctuary to managing breath, muscle relaxation, sounds, aromas, light, nutrition, visualization, writing, and meditation – we arrive at a point of integration. The third and final part of this book is dedicated to consolidating these learnings and cultivating autonomy in our relationship with rest. We begin this final phase with an invitation to gather the threads we have woven so far, to transform the act of falling asleep, often passive or even accidental, into a conscious, intentional, and ritualistic practice. It involves going beyond the isolated application of techniques and starting to orchestrate them harmoniously, learning to read the signals of our own body and using the tools we've acquired as triggers for deep relaxation and serene surrender to sleep. This is the transitional moment where simply "going to sleep" evolves into "falling asleep with awareness," a true mindfulness practice applied at the threshold of rest.

For many people, falling asleep happens almost by chance. We fight sleep until the brink of exhaustion, whether due to work, entertainment, or simply a mind that won't slow down, and eventually "pass out" without any preparation or conscious intention. Or, conversely, we lie in bed hoping sleep will come, but toss and turn, frustrated by the delay, waging an internal battle that only generates more tension. Falling asleep with awareness proposes a radically different approach: facing the moments preceding sleep not as a time of passive waiting or struggle, but as an active period of preparation and transition, nourished by presence and self-compassion.

The first step to falling asleep with awareness is learning to recognize and honor the natural signs of drowsiness our body sends us. Frequent yawning, heavy eyes, difficulty concentrating, a feeling of heaviness in the limbs – these are not signs of weakness to be fought with more caffeine or willpower, but gentle invitations from our organism indicating that the time to begin the disengagement process has arrived. Instead of ignoring these signals or trying to postpone them, we can learn to use them as conscious triggers to start our nightly ritual. Upon noticing the first yawns, instead of opening another browser tab or turning on the television, we can interpret this as: "Ah, my body is telling me it needs rest. It's time to start preparing." This simple shift in attitude, from resistance to acceptance, already initiates the relaxation process.

Based on the body's signals, we begin our personalized nightly ritual, now not as a series of tasks to complete, but as a fluid sequence of practices leading us progressively to a state of greater calm. Here, we integrate the tools learned in previous chapters. Perhaps we start by dimming the ambient lights (light hygiene), putting on soft music or nature sounds (sounds and silences), and having a calming tea (nutrition). Then, we might dedicate a few minutes to therapeutic writing to release the day's worries, or to light reading. Next, perhaps a warm bath with a few drops of lavender (aromatherapy and temperature), followed by a few minutes of gentle stretching or progressive muscle relaxation in bed. And finally, a few minutes of conscious breathing or guided meditation to calm the mind and anchor attention in the present. The order and combination of practices are personal, but the intention is to create a flow that gradually takes us from a state of external activity to a state of internal quietude.

The focus is not on the perfect execution of each technique, but on the presence and intention we bring to each step. We are consciously choosing to disconnect from the outside world and turn inward, caring for our body and mind in preparation for sacred rest. It's an act of respect for ourselves and our vital need for renewal.

In this process, the integration of body-mind-environment becomes fundamental. We realize how the physical environment (the sleep sanctuary, with its appropriate temperature, textures, lights, sounds, and aromas) directly supports our mental and physical relaxation. We use the body as a tool (through breathing and muscle relaxation) to calm the mind. And we use the mind (through visualization, meditation, and writing) to release emotional tensions and focus on the present. These three pillars – body, mind, and environment – cease to be seen as separate entities and come to be understood as interdependent allies in the disengagement process. Falling asleep with awareness is orchestrating this symphony harmoniously.

This approach radically transforms the experience of going to bed. Instead of lying down and passively (or anxiously) waiting for sleep, we lie down with the intention to relax and surrender. If sleep doesn't come immediately, we don't panic or start fighting. We simply return to our anchors – the breath, bodily sensations, a calming visualization – with kindness and patience. We accept the present moment as it is, knowing that the very act of relaxing deeply is already restorative, even if consciousness is still present. Paradoxically, this acceptance and the absence of effort to "make" sleep happen are often what allow it to arise naturally.

Falling asleep with awareness is ultimately a mindfulness practice applied to the threshold of sleep. It's bringing mindful attention, curiosity, and kindness to a process that normally occurs automatically or conflictually. It's recognizing that how we prepare for sleep profoundly impacts the quality of our rest and, by extension, the quality of our waking life. By replacing accidental or forced falling asleep with intentional falling asleep, nurtured by presence and self-care, we not only improve our nights but also cultivate a more intimate, respectful, and harmonious relationship with ourselves.

This new way of approaching sleep, guided by awareness and intention, also reverses a logic deeply ingrained in our culture: that rest must be earned only as a reward for effort or productivity. When we transform falling asleep into a ritual of care, we stop treating sleep as something we "earn" only after an exhausting day and start seeing it as an essential part of life's natural cycle, as worthy of attention as any task of the day. Sleeping ceases to be the endpoint of a busy routine and becomes a sacred transition, inviting us to pause, silence, and restore – not as an escape, but as presence.

As we develop this new relationship with the act of falling asleep, we also refine our inner listening. We begin to perceive more clearly which elements of our ritual truly nourish us, which techniques have more effect on certain days, and how small choices – like how we turn off the phone or the posture we adopt in bed – significantly influence sleep quality. This process of self-knowledge doesn't require rigidity, but rather an open disposition to observe, experiment, and adjust. Over time, the ritual ceases to be a set of techniques and transforms into a living expression of personal care, constantly evolving.

Sleeping with awareness, therefore, is more than achieving a good night's sleep. It's cultivating an attitude that extends beyond the dark room, influencing how we deal with time, the body, emotions, and the day's limits. By lying down with presence, surrendering without resistance, we not only create conditions for restorative sleep but also open space for a more lucid, gentle, and integrated life. In this simple and profound gesture of turning off the light with intention, we ignite a new way of being with ourselves.

Chapter 23
Sleep as Therapy

The practice of falling asleep with awareness, integrating the various tools we've explored, not only facilitates the transition to rest but also opens doors to a deeper understanding of sleep itself: not just as a passive physiological need, but as a powerful and active therapeutic tool. When we intentionally cultivate quality sleep, it transcends its basic function of physical repair and reveals itself as a fundamental agent in emotional restoration, mental clarity, and strengthening the nervous system. Perceiving sleep through this therapeutic lens is recognizing that, night after night, we have the opportunity to dive into a natural and intrinsic healing process, capable of catalyzing significant changes in our well-being and perception of reality. This chapter invites us to deepen this view, exploring how well-slept nights become an active part of our process of self-healing and personal development.

The therapeutic dimension of sleep first manifests in emotional restoration. As we've seen, sleep, especially the REM phase, plays a crucial role in processing and regulating emotions. Emotional experiences from the day, particularly those with a negative or stressful charge, are reprocessed during

REM sleep in a way that seems to diminish their emotional intensity, allowing us to store them as autobiographical memories without the same burden of distress. It's as if the brain performs a "nightly therapy," helping us digest difficult events and integrate emotional learnings. When sleep is insufficient or fragmented, this process is compromised. Negative emotions can persist more intensely, emotional reactivity increases, and the ability to cope with stress diminishes. Conversely, consistently well-slept nights strengthen our emotional resilience, increase our capacity for empathy, improve our overall mood, and allow us to navigate life's challenges with more balance and serenity. Quality sleep acts as a balm for the soul, smoothing emotional edges and restoring our ability to feel and respond more adaptively.

Mental clarity is another direct therapeutic benefit of restorative sleep. During sleep, the brain performs a real cleanup, eliminating toxic metabolic byproducts that accumulate during wakefulness, including proteins associated with neurodegenerative diseases. Furthermore, as already explored, sleep is fundamental for memory consolidation and learning, organizing information, and strengthening important neural connections. The result of well-slept nights is a clearer, more focused, and efficient mind. Concentration improves, reasoning becomes sharper, decision-making is more considered, and creativity flourishes. For those struggling with mental fog, difficulty concentrating, or feeling cognitively overloaded, optimizing sleep can be one of the most effective interventions. It's as if nightly rest restores the mind's natural capacity to operate with clarity and discernment, functioning as natural cognitive therapy.

Strengthening the nervous system is another crucial facet of therapeutic sleep. Chronic sleep deprivation keeps the sympathetic nervous system (fight-or-flight response) hyperactivated, leading to a state of chronic stress that wears down the body and mind. Quality sleep, on the other hand, allows the parasympathetic nervous system (rest-and-digest response) to predominate, promoting recovery, cellular regeneration, and decreased systemic inflammation. A balanced nervous system is the foundation for physical and mental health. It allows us to respond appropriately to daily stressors without collapsing and return to a state of calm more easily. By cultivating restorative sleep, we are actively nurturing and strengthening our nervous system, making it more resilient and less susceptible to the detrimental effects of chronic stress.

Clinical literature and personal accounts are filled with cases where significant sleep improvement was a determining factor in overcoming states of mental suffering, such as depression, generalized anxiety, and burnout syndrome. Although sleep is not an isolated cure for these complex conditions, optimizing it often alleviates symptoms, increases the effectiveness of other therapies (like psychotherapy or medication), and improves the individual's overall quality of life. Restoring a healthy sleep pattern can break the vicious cycle where insomnia worsens anxiety, which in turn makes sleep difficult. It can restore the energy and motivation needed to engage in pleasurable and therapeutic activities essential for depression recovery. It can alleviate the overwhelming sense of physical and mental exhaustion characteristic of burnout. Viewing sleep improvement as an integral part of mental health treatment is fundamental.

More broadly, sleep cultivated with awareness can act as a catalyst for profound changes in various areas of life. When we are rested and emotionally balanced, our perception of reality tends to be more positive and hopeful. We have more clarity to make important decisions aligned with our values. Our behaviors become less reactive and more intentional. The quality of our interpersonal relationships improves, as we have more patience, empathy, and communication skills. The energy restored by sleep motivates us to pursue new projects, take better care of our physical health, and engage in activities that bring us joy and meaning. In short, sleeping well not only makes us feel better in the moment but also empowers us to build a fuller and more satisfying life.

Therefore, the proposal of this chapter is to expand our view of sleep, recognizing it not just as a prerequisite for minimal functioning, but as an active and powerful therapeutic process we can intentionally cultivate. By applying the learned techniques with awareness and consistency, we are not just managing a symptom (like insomnia), but engaging in a profound practice of self-care that nourishes our body, balances our emotions, clears our mind, and strengthens our nervous system.

This perspective invites us to redefine how we relate to sleep in daily life. Instead of treating it as a biological obligation or a concession made to fatigue, we begin to see it as a space of silent and continuous transformation. The simple act of sleeping converts into a therapeutic practice acting on multiple levels, often without our full awareness of its effects. But it is precisely this subtlety that makes it so potent: behind the apparent repose, there is vast work of physical, emotional, and cognitive reorganization underway, restoring the essential balance for living with more health and fullness.

Just as we care for nutrition or seek movements benefiting the body, we can also commit to sleep as an integral part of our therapeutic journey. This choice begins with small attitudes – like respecting our rhythms, cultivating an environment conducive to rest, or simply lying down more gently – and strengthens as we feel its positive reflections in waking life. Over time, we realize that well-slept nights are not just temporary relief, but fertile ground where self-knowledge, patience, creativity, and the courage to change flourish. Sleep then becomes not an end of the day, but a vital link in the chain of our growth.

Embracing sleep as a therapeutic practice is, ultimately, an invitation to trust the intelligence of one's own body and honor the ancestral wisdom of rest. By welcoming sleep as an active ally in the journey of well-being, we stop resisting rest and begin to surrender, night after night, to a process of regeneration that teaches us, in silence, to live with more lightness and presence.

Chapter 24
Cycles and Seasons

As we recognize sleep as a therapeutic process and a practice of conscious self-care, we open space for an even subtler and more integrated understanding: that our need and patterns of sleep are not static, but dynamic and fluid, influenced by myriad internal and external cycles. Just as nature operates in seasonal rhythms, with periods of expansion and withdrawal, our own body and mind respond to changes in daylight duration, temperature variations, and hormonal flows marking different life phases or monthly cycles. Learning to observe and honor these variations, adapting our practices and expectations instead of fighting against them, is a fundamental step towards cultivating a truly harmonious and sustainable relationship with rest. This chapter invites us to tune into these natural rhythms, understanding sleep as something living and sensitive, to be welcomed with flexibility, respect, and wisdom.

The most evident influence on our sleep patterns is the cycle of seasons, particularly the variation in daylight duration. At latitudes farther from the equator, winters bring longer nights and shorter days, with lower sunlight intensity, while summers present the opposite pattern. Our biological clock is highly sensitive to these changes. Less light exposure during the winter day can lead to less robust or slightly desynchronized melatonin production, potentially resulting in greater daytime sleepiness, lower energy, and, for some people, a tendency to need slightly more nighttime sleep. This is popularly known as "winter blues" or, in more severe cases, Seasonal Affective Disorder (SAD), where lack of light significantly impacts mood and energy levels. Recognizing this natural tendency towards withdrawal during the darker, colder months is important. Instead of fighting it with excess stimulants or self-criticism, we can welcome this need, perhaps adjusting our schedules to allow a bit more rest, intensifying the search for natural light in the morning (even if diffuse), and focusing on restorative practices.

In summer, with longer days and greater light intensity, our biological clock receives a stronger signal for wakefulness. We might naturally feel more energized and need slightly less sleep. However, excessive heat can make falling asleep and staying asleep difficult, requiring adaptations in the bedroom environment, as discussed in the chapter on temperature. Additionally, increased social activity and vacations can lead to more irregular sleep schedules which, if not managed consciously, can lead to "social jet lag" and compromise rest quality, even if the total sleep need is slightly lower. The key is finding balance, harnessing the season's energy without sacrificing regularity and sleep hygiene practices.

Temperature changes between seasons also require adaptations. Winter cold can make it harder to get out of a warm bed in the morning or cause discomfort if the room isn't adequately heated. Summer heat, as mentioned, can be a major sleep disruptor. Learning to adjust the room environment, sleepwear, and bedding according to the season is essential for maintaining the thermal comfort necessary for good sleep. It's a constant dance of fine-tuning, listening to the body's needs in response to weather conditions.

Besides external seasonal cycles, we are subject to internal cycles, like hormonal ones. In women of reproductive age, the menstrual cycle brings significant hormonal fluctuations that can impact sleep. For example, in the premenstrual phase, the drop in progesterone levels (a hormone with relaxing effects) and cramps or discomfort can make sleep difficult. During pregnancy, hormonal changes, physical discomfort, and anxiety can drastically alter sleep patterns. In menopause, decreased estrogen and progesterone levels are often associated with night sweats, insomnia, and other sleep disorders. Recognizing these hormonal influences allows us to approach them with more understanding and seek specific strategies for each phase, whether through lifestyle adjustments, complementary therapies, or medical follow-up when necessary.

Different life stages also bring distinct sleep needs. Infants and children need many hours of sleep for physical and neurological development. Teenagers undergo a natural shift in their biological clock making them more nocturnal, needing to sleep and wake later – something that often conflicts with school schedules.

Adults generally need 7 to 9 hours of sleep per night, but this need can vary individually. Elderly individuals may experience lighter, more fragmented sleep with more nighttime awakenings, although the total sleep need doesn't drastically decrease. Understanding these age-related changes helps adjust expectations and adapt sleep hygiene strategies for each phase.

Times of increased stress, illness, major transitions, or emotionally demanding phases also increase our need for rest. When going through a difficult period, be it a loss, a job change, a health challenge, or simply a period of high emotional demand, the body and mind need more time to recover and process experiences. At these times, it's crucial to honor this increased need for sleep, instead of trying to maintain the usual pace. Allowing yourself more rest, being kinder to yourself, and intensifying self-care practices (including the relaxation techniques learned) is an act of wisdom and self-compassion. Sleep acts as a fundamental therapeutic resource during these phases, helping us navigate them with more resilience.

The invitation of this chapter is for you to become an attentive observer of your own cycles and the seasonal and personal influences on your sleep. Maintain flexibility in your routine and expectations. Realize that your sleep won't be exactly the same every night or every season, and that's normal. Learn to adapt your rituals and practices according to the needs of the moment. Perhaps you need more relaxation time in winter, or extra care with temperature in summer. Perhaps you need to be more patient with yourself during certain phases of the menstrual cycle or during stressful periods. Understanding sleep as something dynamic, sensitive, and responsive to the rhythms of life and nature frees us from the rigidity and frustration of trying to achieve a perfect, immutable pattern.

This organic view of sleep, rooted in listening to natural rhythms, offers a gentler and more sustainable path to self-care. Instead of trying to shape rest to a fixed ideal or external model, we begin to live it as a continuous dialogue with the body, the environment, and the seasons of life. This attentive listening doesn't require advanced technical knowledge, just presence and curiosity: how am I sleeping this week? What signals has my body been giving me? What has changed in me or around me that might be influencing this cycle? This kind of attention transforms the practice of sleep into a sensitive art, where small observations lead to great discoveries about our own needs.

By making space for this flexibility, we recognize that true self-care is not control, but conscious adaptation. This implies accepting that there will be phases when we sleep more, others when sleep will be lighter, transition periods when the body will demand new forms of support. The important thing is to be available to adjust, reconfigure, and above all, welcome. This fluidity also allows us to cultivate a less anxious relationship with sleep: we understand that fluctuations are not failures, but natural expressions of life in motion. This understanding protects us from frustration and strengthens us with a deeper sense of connection to who we are – cyclical beings in a world that pulses in cycles.

In this way, sleeping well ceases to be a rigid goal and becomes a continuous dance with the rhythms of nature and our own existence. By recognizing and respecting these variations, we build a more authentic and resilient rest – a sleep that accompanies our history, our phases, our internal and external seasons. And it is precisely in this meeting between flexibility and presence that the wisdom of truly restorative sleep resides.

Chapter 25
The Inner Journey

As we learn to embrace the cyclical nature of sleep and adapt our practices with flexibility and respect, our relationship with rest begins to transcend the mere management of habits and environments. We enter a deeper domain, where the act of sleeping reveals itself not only as a physiological necessity or a therapeutic tool, but as a true inner journey, a nocturnal voyage of reconnection with the subtler layers of our being. This chapter invites us to explore this symbolic and sensitive dimension of sleep, to perceive it as a dive into the vast ocean of the unconscious, where dreams, fragmented sensations, and unexpected insights can emerge as precious messages from our own soul. Valuing the time of sleep as a sacred space for encountering oneself expands our consciousness and enriches our journey of self-knowledge, revealing that sleeping well is also rediscovering oneself in depth each night.

The idea of sleep as a journey is not new; it permeates mythologies, spiritual traditions, and depth psychology. When we fall asleep, the rational and vigilant consciousness dominating our waking state recedes, allowing other forms of perception and processing to surface. The veil between the conscious and unconscious becomes thinner, and we are invited to navigate inner landscapes reflecting our fears, desires, unresolved conflicts, and latent potentials. Dreams, with their often illogical, symbolic, and emotionally charged language, are the most evident manifestation of this nocturnal activity of the psyche. They can confront us with shadow aspects we avoid during the day, offer creative solutions to problems that seemed insoluble, or connect us with universal archetypes and sources of inner wisdom. Learning to welcome dreams, even unsettling ones, as messengers from our inner world is an essential part of this journey.

But the inner journey of sleep is not limited to the narrative dreams predominantly occurring in the REM phase. Even in deeper sleep stages (NREM), or in moments of transition between wakefulness and sleep (hypnagogia) and between sleep and waking (hypnopompia), we can access fragments of images, intense bodily sensations, loose words, or sudden insights that seem to spring from a place beyond the rational mind. They are echoes of the unconscious, flashes of intuition, bodily responses to healing and integration processes occurring at deep levels while we rest. We often dismiss these experiences as irrelevant or "all in the head," but if we learn to pay attention to them, with curiosity and openness, they can offer valuable clues about our inner state and deepest needs.

Valuing sleep as an inner journey begins with intention. As we prepare for sleep, we can include in our ritual the intention to be open to messages from our unconscious, to welcome our dreams and nocturnal sensations as part of our process of growth and self-knowledge. We can ask for clarity on a specific issue or simply adopt an attitude of receptivity to whatever emerges from our inner world during the night. This simple shift in attitude transforms sleep from a passive event into an active opportunity for inner dialogue.

Upon waking, even before opening your eyes or getting up, reserve a few moments to remain in silence, trying to recall fragments of dreams or sensations still present. Keep a notebook and pen beside the bed (as suggested in the chapter on nightly writing and detailed further in the next on the sleep diary) to immediately jot down any memory, however strange or fleeting it seems. Don't try to interpret or analyze immediately; just record the images, emotions, characters, or words that come to mind. The act of recording honors the experience and helps bring it into consciousness.

Integrating these nocturnal perceptions into daily life is where the inner journey gains practical meaning. Throughout the day, or in moments of reflection, return to your notes. What emotions did the dream or sensation evoke? Are there parallels with situations or feelings you are currently experiencing? Is there a recurring image or symbol? Instead of seeking literal interpretations or resorting to generic dream dictionaries, trust your own intuition and the associations that arise for you. Ask yourself: "What does this image or sensation mean *to me*, in my current context?" Sometimes the meaning might be clear; other times, it may remain a mystery or reveal itself gradually over time. The important thing is to maintain an open and respectful dialogue with these contents, recognizing them as authentic expressions of your psyche.

We can also use simple reflection exercises or creative practices to deepen this integration. Drawing or painting a striking dream image can release associated emotions and reveal new meanings. Writing an imaginary dialogue with a dream character can bring clarity to internal conflicts. Meditating on the predominant feeling of a dream can help understand its central message. Sharing a significant dream with a trusted friend or therapist (if applicable) can also offer new perspectives. The goal is not to dissect the dream intellectually, but to feel its impact and allow it to inform our waking life in some way.

Perceiving sleep as an inner journey helps us cultivate a richer, multidimensional relationship with rest. It ceases to be just a period of physical inactivity and becomes a time of profound psychic and spiritual activity, a sacred space where we can meet forgotten or unknown parts of ourselves, process experiences, release blockages, and access sources of creativity and wisdom. This perspective infuses the act of sleeping with a sense of purpose and reverence, motivating us to take even better care of the conditions allowing this journey to happen as peacefully and restoratively as possible. By embracing sleep as this nocturnal opportunity for diving into our inner universe, we realize that each night is a chance to be reborn slightly more conscious, more integrated, and more connected with the totality of our being. The quality of our sleep comes to be measured not only by the feeling of physical rest in the morning but also by the richness of perceptions and insights we bring back from this silent voyage.

As this practice deepens, sleep transforms into fertile territory where the unconscious, far from being a feared enigma or dark zone, becomes an ally in the growth process. What emerges during the night—intense dreams, fleeting images, or even just restorative silence—comes to be valued as an extension of consciousness itself, a symbolic language needing to be heard with respect and sensitivity. Over time, this constant listening develops an intimacy with the inner world that isn't restricted just to sleep time but radiates into the day, influencing decisions, relationships, and how we experience existence itself.

This nocturnal journey also teaches that we don't need to have all the answers upon waking. The inner journey of sleep is not a map with fixed destinations, but a process of living navigation respecting the mysteries of the unconscious. Not everything will be clear, not everything will be immediately understood—and that's not a problem, but an intrinsic part of the depth of this encounter. The beauty lies precisely in allowing these experiences to flow, without demanding control, without needing immediate results. Each night, we expand the internal space so that listening, presence, and acceptance guide us more confidently through the invisible territories of being. By caring for sleep with this loving and curious attention, we discover it offers us not just rest, but direction. It's a daily return to essence, a constant reminder that there is, within us, a vast and wise universe waiting to be explored. And the more we open ourselves to this journey, the more whole we awaken—not just because we slept well, but because we traveled deep, and returned bringing a little more of ourselves back.

Chapter 26
Sleep Diary

The journey of self-knowledge and transformation of our relationship with sleep, which we have tread throughout these chapters, gains a practical and powerful ally in the form of a sleep diary. We briefly mentioned the importance of recording observations during personal diagnosis and noting dreams and insights from the inner journey. Now, we deepen this idea, proposing the creation of a diary specifically dedicated to tracking our sleep patterns, related habits, and subjective perception of rest quality. Far from being another bureaucratic task, the sleep diary, when used with intention and curiosity, transforms into a dynamic tool for self-regulation, a mirror reflecting our progress and challenges, and a valuable instrument for clearly identifying what works and what needs adjustment in our quest for more restorative nights. It's an act of commitment to ourselves, a tangible record of our journey towards healing and well-being.

Keeping a sleep diary helps bring objectivity to an area often dominated by vague perceptions or inaccurate memories. How many hours did we really sleep? What time did we go to bed and get up? Did we have nighttime awakenings? How did we feel upon waking?

Relying solely on memory can be misleading. Systematically recording this information over days and weeks allows us to visualize patterns that would otherwise go unnoticed. It helps us correlate our daytime and nighttime habits with the resulting sleep quality, revealing important connections between our actions and their consequences for rest. For example, we might notice that on nights we used screens late, our sleep was more restless, or that after a particularly stressful day, we had more difficulty falling asleep. Or, conversely, we might find that introducing a consistent nightly ritual or a specific relaxation technique coincided with an improved feeling of rest in the morning.

What to record in a sleep diary? The structure can be simple and adapted to your needs, but some key elements are generally recommended to provide a useful overview. Ideally, the diary would have two parts: one filled out at night, before sleep, and another in the morning, right after waking up.

In the nightly section, you can record: the time you are going to bed; a brief description of your physical and emotional state (tired, relaxed, anxious, agitated?); what activities you did in the last hour before bed (your nightly ritual); consumption of substances that might affect sleep in the last few hours (caffeine, alcohol, medications); and perhaps a brief note about significant events or stress levels of the day. Recording this information at night helps create awareness about factors preceding sleep.

In the morning section, right upon waking, note: the time you woke up; an estimate of the total time you believe you slept; the number of nighttime awakenings you recall and, if possible, the duration or reason; the overall perceived sleep quality (you can use a scale of 1 to 5, for example, or words like "poor," "fair," "good," "excellent"); how you feel upon waking (rested, groggy, energetic, tired?); and any dreams you can remember, even if just fragments or emotions (as explored in the previous chapter). Filling this part out in the morning, while sensations are still fresh, provides valuable data about the night's outcome.

To make the diary practice more pleasant and less burdensome, choose a notebook that appeals to you visually and a comfortable pen. Keep it beside the bed for easy access. Don't worry about writing lengthy texts; short, objective notes are sufficient. Use symbols, scales, or keywords if you prefer. The important thing is consistency. Try filling it out daily for at least two weeks to start identifying patterns. After this initial period, you can choose to keep it continuously or use it periodically, especially when implementing new changes or going through phases of greater difficulty with sleep.

Transforming the diary into a pleasant practice involves seeing it not as an obligation, but as an act of curiosity and self-care. View it as a dialogue with yourself, a space to investigate your own experience gently. Celebrate the small improvements you observe. Use colors, drawings, or inspiring quotes if that motivates you. The diary is yours and should serve your needs.

Besides identifying patterns and correlating habits with results, the sleep diary is a powerful tool for tracking changes over time. As you implement the techniques and strategies learned in this course, you can use the diary to objectively monitor their effects. Is nightly meditation helping reduce awakenings? Did changing the bedroom lighting improve the morning feeling of rest? The diary provides concrete feedback, allowing you to adjust your practices based on evidence from your own experience, rather than just assumptions. It also serves as a record of your progress, which can be very motivating, especially in moments when the journey feels more challenging. Looking back and seeing how far you've come reinforces your commitment and confidence in your ability to transform your relationship with sleep.

Periodically reflecting on the information recorded in the diary is fundamental. Set aside time each week, for example, to review your notes. Look for trends, connections, and insights. What seems to be working well? What needs more attention or adjustment? This reflection transforms raw data into practical wisdom, guiding your next choices and actions.

In essence, the sleep diary is much more than a simple data log. It's an instrument of self-knowledge, a catalyst for conscious change, and a testament to your commitment to the sleep healing process. This simple yet profoundly transformative practice reveals the power in making visible what normally goes unnoticed. The act of recording, night after night, details of sleep and the sensations accompanying it invites us out of automaticity and into a state of active, sensitive observation. By writing them down, our patterns cease to be mere repeated behaviors and gain shape, history, and meaning. Gradually, we discover the diary is not just a mirror, but also a compass—it shows us where we are going and how we are walking. And, in many cases, it shows us that true transformation begins precisely with the willingness to look honestly at daily experience.

Over time, writing this diary becomes almost a meditative ritual. Instead of a mechanical task, it becomes a moment of connection—a brief but significant interval where we turn our gaze inward and listen to the body more attentively. We notice that certain days demand more silence, that particular practices repeat because they work, or that there are predictable relapses during weeks of higher tension. This continuous listening develops not only awareness but also autonomy: we stop depending solely on external formulas and learn to respond to our real needs, creatively and gently. The diary, in this sense, is also a process of emotional education, as it teaches us to name what we feel and care for it with more maturity.

Ultimately, keeping a sleep diary is much more than collecting information: it's sustaining, with patience and tenderness, a listening space where body, mind, and unconscious can manifest. It's reaffirming, day after day, the commitment to care for rest as a sacred act of presence. And when we look back and leaf through these pages, we see not just data—we see our own history being written with more consciousness, depth, and clarity. In this continuous record, we are simultaneously witnesses and protagonists of the journey we undertake towards a more integral, restorative, and true sleep.

Chapter 27
Sleep and Creativity

Throughout this journey, we have explored sleep from various perspectives: as a biological need, a pillar of health, a cyclical process, a state influenced by habits and environment, an inner journey, and even a therapeutic tool. Now, we add another fascinating layer to this multifaceted understanding: the intimate and powerful connection between deep rest and the flourishing of creativity. Countering the limiting belief that sleep is time lost to productivity, a view increasingly supported by science and the experience of countless artists, scientists, and innovators emerges: the resting brain is not inactive, but engaged in crucial processes that consolidate ideas, stimulate unexpected connections, and favor the emergence of creative solutions. This chapter invites us to see sleep as a strategic ally of our creative potential, a fertile space where the mind, free from the constraints of linear waking logic, can weave new possibilities and present us with valuable insights upon awakening.

The idea that sleep nurtures creativity is not just a romantic intuition; it finds basis in the neurological processes occurring while we sleep. During sleep, especially in NREM (slow-wave sleep) and REM phases, the brain is actively working on reorganizing and consolidating information acquired during the day. In NREM sleep, short-term memories are transferred from the hippocampus to the neocortex, where they are stored more permanently and integrated with existing knowledge. This process strengthens memories and frees up space in the hippocampus for new learning the next day. REM sleep, with its high brain activity and vivid dreams, seems to play a fundamental role in forming new and unexpected associations between seemingly unrelated pieces of information. The reduced influence of the neurotransmitter norepinephrine during REM allows the brain to explore more distant and less obvious connections, an essential ingredient for creative thinking and "outside-the-box" problem-solving.

It's as if the brain, during sleep, performs a kind of internal "brainstorming." It revisits the day's problems and challenges, but in a more fluid and less structured way than in wakefulness. Neural networks reconfigure, testing new combinations and perspectives. Information stored in different brain areas can be connected in surprising ways, leading to insights that wouldn't occur under the filter of logic and criticism prevalent when we're awake. This process of nocturnal incubation explains why we often wake up with the solution to a problem that tormented us the day before, or with a new and original idea that seems to have appeared "out of nowhere." Sleep not only consolidates what we already know but also helps us see things in a new light, find hidden patterns, and generate new syntheses.

History is replete with anecdotal examples illustrating this connection. German chemist August Kekulé reportedly discovered the ring structure of the benzene molecule after dreaming of a snake biting its own tail. Inventor Elias Howe credited a nightmare with the idea for the design of the sewing machine needle. Composer Paul McCartney claims the melody for the song "Yesterday" came to him in a dream. Artists like Salvador Dalí used techniques to access the hypnagogic state (between wakefulness and sleep) seeking surreal images for their works. Scientists often report having epiphanies about complex problems after a night's sleep or upon waking. These stories, though not rigorous scientific proof in themselves, point to a universal human experience: the recognition that deep rest can be a powerful catalyst for inspiration and innovation.

Understanding this relationship invites us to rethink our approach to productivity and problem-solving. Instead of forcing the mind to find solutions through continuous effort and sleep deprivation, we can learn to trust the power of rest as an integral part of the creative process. When faced with a creative block or a complex problem, "sleeping on it" is not an act of procrastination, but an intelligent strategy. By allowing the brain to work in the background during sleep, we increase the chances that new connections and insights will emerge. This requires a mindset shift, abandoning the idea that creativity depends solely on conscious effort and embracing the wisdom of the unconscious manifested in repose.

We can even actively cultivate this creative potential of sleep. Before sleeping, we can dedicate a few minutes to reflect on a problem or creative question we wish to explore, without pressure to find an immediate answer. Simply plant the seed in the mind, intending for the unconscious to work on it during the night. Keeping a notebook and pen beside the bed, as already suggested, becomes even more crucial in this context. The moment of awakening, especially that transition phase between sleep and full wakefulness (hypnopompic state), is often a period of great mental fluidity, where ideas and images from the dream world are still accessible. Immediately noting any thoughts, ideas, dream fragments, or solutions that arise at this moment can capture precious insights before they dissipate in the light of waking consciousness. Don't censor or judge what comes up; just record it.

We can extend this practice to the first moments after waking. Instead of immediately grabbing the phone or diving into the day's tasks, reserve a few minutes to remain quiet, perhaps still in bed, and allow the mind to wander freely. Use this fertile time to record creative thoughts, sketch ideas, freewrite, or plan projects with the renewed clarity sleep provides. Treat this waking moment as a sacred space for creativity, a gift offered by nightly rest.

This perspective transforms our view of sleep. It ceases to be merely a period of physical recovery and also becomes an incubator of ideas, a laboratory for unexpected connections, and a source of personal and professional innovation. Recognizing and cultivating the connection between sleep and creativity aligns us with a healthier and more sustainable form of productivity, where rest is not seen as an obstacle, but as an essential ingredient. It's understanding that by honoring our need for repose, we are also nurturing our ability to create, solve problems, and bring new ideas into the world.

As we incorporate this wisdom into our routine, we realize that creative sleep is not the privilege of inspired geniuses, but a possibility within reach of anyone willing to listen to the natural rhythm of their mind. It's not just about sleeping more, but sleeping with intention, preparing the mental ground before rest, making space for the unexpected upon waking. By accepting that part of our deepest work happens in silence, while we dream, we open doors to a more fluid and intuitive creativity, less driven by control and more anchored in the trust that the mind knows how to navigate territories beyond our conscious command.

In this sense, valuing sleep is also an act of creative humility. It's admitting there is a silent intelligence within us that reorganizes, combines, unfolds, and reinterprets lived experiences, even when our will is suspended. Sleep connects us with less accessible layers of the mind—fertile zones where symbols, emotions, and memories intertwine, revealing unsuspected paths. By cultivating this bond, we begin to perceive creativity not as a sporadic flash, but as a continuous process, fueled by both doing and resting, by effort and surrender, by wakefulness and dreaming.

Thus, creativity reveals itself as a cycle completed in rest. Each well-slept night can be the soil where ideas germinate that will transform our next day. Honoring this process respects the very nature of the human mind, made of rhythm, pause, and flow. Sleep, far from distancing us from the creative world, immerses us in its depths—and it is from there, from dreamlike silence and free associations, that ideas emerge which illuminate, transform, and advance.

Chapter 28
Mini-Sleep Retreats

The idea of "sleep tourism," previously introduced as a growing trend in specialized destinations, might seem distant or inaccessible to many. However, the essence behind this concept – the intentional creation of a period and space dedicated exclusively to deep rest and reconnecting with oneself – can be adapted and experienced in the comfort of our own home. This chapter introduces the practice of "mini-sleep retreats": specific immersion experiences in rest that we can plan and carry out at home, taking advantage of weekends, holidays, or even a single day off, aiming to restore vital energy, deepen the learned relaxation practices, and offer the body and mind an intensive break from daily demands. It's a democratic and accessible way to experience the benefits of a sleep-focused retreat without needing to travel, transforming our home into a true nocturnal recovery spa.

We live at a pace that often pushes us to the brink of exhaustion. Even with the implementation of sleep hygiene habits and nightly rituals, accumulated stress and fatigue can persist. Mini-sleep retreats emerge as a complementary strategy, offering an opportunity to "reset" the system more concentratedly. Instead of waiting for annual vacations to slow down, we can periodically incorporate these restorative breaks into our calendar, recognizing that intensive moments of rest are as important as daily sleep for maintaining long-term health and well-being. It's a proactive investment in our own vitality.

How to plan and structure a mini-sleep retreat at home? The first step is intention and planning. Choose a period – it could be a long weekend, a Saturday and Sunday, or even a single day when you can disconnect from external obligations. Communicate your intention to the people living with you, explaining the importance of this withdrawal time and asking for cooperation to minimize interruptions and noise. The idea is to create a bubble of tranquility within your own home.

The main focus of the mini-retreat is the radical reduction of external stimuli and maximizing time dedicated to rest and restorative practices. Disconnect as much as possible from the digital world: silence notifications, avoid checking emails or social media, and consider keeping your phone stored in another room most of the time. Also, reduce exposure to news or content that might generate anxiety or mental agitation. The goal is to create a space of silence not only external but also internal.

Transform your bedroom (and, if possible, other areas of the house) into a true sanctuary, intensifying the care we've already discussed. Ensure total darkness, silence (using earplugs or white noise if necessary), pleasant temperature, and maximum comfort in bed. Use aromatherapy with relaxing essential oils. Prepare the environment so it invites rest at any time of day or night.

Create a simple and flexible schedule for your retreat, without the rigidity of a work agenda, but with a structure guiding your activities. Prioritize sleep: allow yourself to sleep more hours than usual if you feel the need, without guilt. Naps during the day are also welcome if the body asks for them. The goal is to follow your body's natural rhythm, allowing it to recover accumulated sleep debt.

Incorporate various relaxation practices learned throughout the day. Dedicate longer times to meditation, conscious breathing, or progressive muscle relaxation. Take prolonged warm baths with salts and oils. Read inspiring books or listen to extremely calm music. Practice restorative yoga or gentle stretches. Do guided visualizations. The retreat is an opportunity to deepen these practices without time pressure.

Nutrition during the mini-retreat should also be light, nutritious, and favorable to relaxation. Avoid heavy foods, stimulants, or alcohol. Hydrate well with water and calming teas. Prepare simple meals or opt for foods requiring little preparation, so as not to expend excessive energy in the kitchen. The focus is on gently nourishing the body.

Allow yourself moments of quietude and contemplation. Sit silently observing nature through the window, practice therapeutic writing to process emotions, or simply do nothing, allowing the mind to rest without needing to fill every moment with activity.

Boredom, in this context, can be a portal to deep relaxation and creativity.

The duration of the mini-retreat can vary. A full weekend (from Friday evening to Sunday evening) can offer deeper restoration. But even a single day dedicated to these practices can make a significant difference in your energy and stress levels. What matters is the quality of immersion and the intention placed on this period.

At the end of your mini-retreat, observe how you feel. You will likely notice a greater sense of calm, mental clarity, renewed energy, and a deeper connection with yourself. This experience reinforces the perception of the therapeutic power of rest and the importance of prioritizing it not only daily but also through these intensive, intentional breaks.

Mini-sleep retreats at home are, therefore, a practical and accessible way to apply the principles of sleep tourism without leaving home. They teach us that we don't need to wait for ideal external conditions or expensive trips to deeply care for our rest. We can create oases of tranquility and restoration within our own daily lives.

By integrating mini-sleep retreats as part of a conscious self-care routine, we begin to view rest not as sporadic relief, but as an active practice of regeneration. These moments become powerful reminders that life doesn't have to be lived in constant acceleration. Each intentional pause helps us reconnect with a more authentic rhythm, where listening to the body and respecting its limits becomes a priority. This deep listening, cultivated in silence and repose, leads us back to the essential—an inner space where clarity and serenity have a chance to flourish.

The strength of mini-retreats lies not just in the absence of stimuli, but in creating an environment that invites self-acceptance. They allow us access to a more receptive state, where the mind slows down and opens to subtle perceptions, neglected feelings, and even answers that previously seemed unattainable. Unlike exhaustive productivity demanding constant effort, this deep rest shows us there is power in surrender, pause, and gentleness. We discover, thus, that restoring oneself is also an act of courage—of stepping out of automaticity to, however briefly, inhabit life with more presence and lightness. It is in this simple and transformative gesture that mini-retreats find their true beauty: they remind us that rest doesn't need to be negotiated, postponed, or idealized. It can be lived, here and now, as a reunion with what is most vital. Creating this space within the home is an act of care for the body, mind, and spirit—a loving return to one's own inner home.

Chapter 29
Sleep Tourism

We revisit in this chapter a concept introduced earlier, "sleep tourism," but now with a deeper look and broader perspective. If before we presented it as an emerging trend, now we explore it as a consolidated and expanding field, with its own destinations, therapies, structures, and philosophies, reflecting a significant shift in how we view rest and well-being in our travels and lives overall. Delving into the universe of sleep tourism is not just about knowing specialized hotels and spas, but understanding a movement that places restorative rest at the center of the experience, inviting us to consider investing in our sleep as a legitimate form of leisure, self-care, and personal development. More than a market niche, sleep tourism can become a life philosophy, inspiring us to transform not just specific trips, but any journey, into an opportunity to cultivate restorative rest.

The sleep tourism landscape today is vast and diverse. Luxury hotels in major urban centers and secluded resorts amidst nature are investing heavily in creating environments and programs far beyond just a quiet room. We find suites designed by sleep experts, featuring circadian lighting systems mimicking the solar cycle, high-tech mattresses and pillows with customizable firmness and temperature options, pillow menus with different heights and materials, and state-of-the-art soundproofing. Some offer "sleep concierges," trained professionals to assist guests in optimizing their rest, from choosing the ideal pillow to suggesting relaxing teas or scheduling therapies.

Night spas and wellness programs focused on sleep are also multiplying. Beyond traditional relaxing massages, we find innovative therapies like flotation in sensory deprivation tanks (drastically reducing external stimuli), hyperbaric chambers (increasing oxygenation and potentially promoting relaxation), infrared light therapies (which may help reduce pain and inflammation), and biofeedback or neurofeedback sessions (training self-regulation of physiological responses and brainwaves associated with relaxation). Workshops on sleep hygiene, meditation and breathing techniques, and consultations with nutritionists or sleep specialist doctors complement the offerings, providing guests with practical tools to take home.

Sleep retreats represent an even deeper immersion. Usually located in tranquil natural settings, these retreats offer multi-day programs fully dedicated to reprogramming sleep habits and restoring vital energy. They combine optimized accommodations, healthy food, daily practices of yoga, meditation, and mindfulness, body therapies, educational workshops, and crucially, an environment free from digital distractions and daily stress. The proposal is to create a safe and welcoming space where participants can disconnect from the outside world, reconnect with themselves, and relearn the art of resting deeply, often with the guidance of a multidisciplinary team of experts.

This growing sophistication of sleep tourism reflects an increasing demand for effective solutions to the epidemic of sleep deprivation and chronic stress plaguing modern society. People are realizing that investing in their rest is not a whim, but a fundamental necessity for health, happiness, and productivity. In this context, considering a trip focused on sleep ceases to be seen as eccentric and starts being viewed as an intelligent investment in oneself, a form of leisure bringing lasting benefits to all areas of life. Just as we invest in education, health, or professional development, investing in our sleep through a dedicated tourism experience can be equally valuable and transformative.

However, the philosophy of sleep tourism transcends the need to travel to specific destinations. The deeper invitation is for us to reflect: how can we transform *every* trip, whether for work or leisure, into an experience that also nurtures our rest? This involves taking the awareness and practices we have cultivated with us. When booking a hotel, we can research room quality, request a quiet floor, or bring our own "sleep kits" with masks, earplugs, favorite essential oils, or a small white noise generator. We can maintain, as much as possible, a regular sleep routine, even when away from home. We can take advantage of the trip to disconnect a bit more from work and social media, especially at night. We can make more conscious food choices, avoiding excesses that impair sleep. We can use free time to practice relaxation, meditation, or simply contemplate the scenery.

This approach transforms travel from a potential sleep disruptor into an opportunity to practice self-care in a new context. It requires planning and intention, but the benefits of returning from a trip feeling genuinely rested, rather than even more exhausted, are immense. We begin to view sleep not as something to be sacrificed for the "full experience" of the trip, but as an integral and essential part of that experience.

In this broadened perspective, sleep tourism becomes less about the destination and more about the attitude. It's a life philosophy integrating respect for rest into all our activities, recognizing that our ability to enjoy any experience – be it a business meeting, a museum visit, or a day at the beach – is directly influenced by the quality of our repose.

This paradigm shift invites a profound review of how we relate to time, the body, and the very idea of pleasure. Sleep tourism, unlike trips driven by frantic schedules, proposes a return to the essential: living well begins with sleeping well. By choosing destinations or creating experiences that prioritize rest, we are taking an active stance of care for our mental and emotional health, rescuing a sensitivity often muffled by the constant urgency of daily life. More than a passing trend, this movement reflects a collective desire for reconciliation with life's natural rhythms.

Furthermore, realizing that rest can be a legitimate source of pleasure and learning broadens our notion of well-being. It's not just about sleeping more hours, but about qualifying that time with awareness and presence. Sleep tourism inspires us to imagine travel experiences that are transformative precisely because they return us to ourselves, with more clarity, lightness, and vitality. It reminds us that true luxury often lies in simplicity—in a quiet room, a contemplative sunset, a body finally finding deep repose. This valuation of rest as an essential part of living well is, in itself, a revolutionary gesture.

By adopting this philosophy, we carry a new lens through which to view the world and plan our relationship with it. No matter the destination: what changes is how we choose to traverse it. Sleep tourism, in this sense, not only offers new ways to travel but also proposes a new way of being—more respectful of the body's limits, more attentive to internal needs, and, above all, more generous with one's own time.

Chapter 30
The House of Sleep

Our journey towards restorative sleep and a more balanced life has led us to explore our inner world – biology, habits, beliefs – and optimize our most intimate resting space: the bedroom, transformed into a sanctuary. However, the environment's influence on our well-being is not limited to the four walls where we sleep. The general atmosphere of our home, the rhythms we cultivate in common spaces, and how we interact with the people we share our home with also play a crucial role in our ability to slow down, relax, and ultimately sleep well. This chapter proposes an expansion of the sanctuary concept, inviting us to apply the principles of tranquility, organization, and awareness cultivated in the bedroom to our entire home. It's about creating not just a sleep room, but a "house of sleep," a home where the culture of deceleration and respect for rest permeates all environments and routines, recognizing that the quality of our nights begins to be woven long before we reach the bed, in the very fabric of our daily lives and the environment where it unfolds.

If the bedroom is the heart of our rest, the entire house is the body supporting it. A chaotic, noisy, overly lit house, or one marked by stressful family routines, especially during evening hours, can undermine the best efforts to create a tranquil refuge in the bedroom. The contrast between a sanctuary-bedroom and a chaos-house can be so great that the transition to relaxation becomes difficult. On the other hand, a home where a general atmosphere of calm, order, and respect for individual rhythms prevails greatly facilitates the disengagement process and prepares the ground for more peaceful sleep for all its inhabitants.

Applying sanctuary principles to the entire house begins with managing light and sound in common areas, especially at night. Just as in the bedroom, reducing lighting intensity in living rooms, kitchens, and hallways in the hours leading up to everyone's bedtime helps collectively signal that the day is ending. Swapping bright bulbs for dimmer, warm-toned options, using lamps instead of ceiling lights, and encouraging reduced use of bright screens in shared spaces contributes to a more relaxing atmosphere. Similarly, being mindful of noise levels is fundamental. Loud conversations, high-volume televisions or music, noise from appliances, or noisy activities late at night can disturb not only those already trying to sleep but also those trying to relax and prepare for rest. Cultivating collective awareness about noise impact and establishing agreements on quiet hours or headphone use can make a big difference in the home's sound harmony.

Organization and the absence of visual clutter in common spaces also contribute to an overall sense of calm. A tidy living room, a clean kitchen, and an organized entryway invite tranquility, while chaotic environments can generate a subliminal sense of stress and pending tasks. Encouraging all family members to collaborate in maintaining order, creating simple organization systems, and establishing tidying routines helps create a physical environment supporting everyone's mental well-being. A visually serene home is a home more conducive to relaxation.

Creating family routines respecting the need for nighttime deceleration is another crucial aspect. If evenings at home are marked by arguments, last-minute school or work activities, or constant commotion, it becomes difficult for any family member to enter a state of relaxation. It's important to discuss and jointly establish routines favoring calm in the final hours of the day. This might include setting a cut-off time for more demanding activities, encouraging shared relaxing activities (like reading aloud, quiet board games, or simply talking calmly), and creating family rituals signaling the transition to a period of lower activity, like a shared light snack or a moment of gratitude together.

Coexistence and respect for individual spaces and needs within the home are also fundamental. In shared homes, open and respectful dialogue about sleep habits and everyone's needs is essential. Understanding that different people may have different schedules or sensitivities (to noise, light, etc.) and seeking solutions accommodating everyone's needs promotes an environment of greater harmony and less friction. Establishing clear rules about using common spaces at night, respecting the need for quiet of those already retired, and demonstrating empathy for other family members' sleep difficulties strengthens bonds and contributes to a more supportive and peaceful domestic environment.

Re-evaluating our relationship with home through the lens of sleep invites us to perceive the house not just as a physical shelter, but as a living ecosystem directly influencing our rhythm and well-being. Every choice we make about organization, lighting, sounds, and routines within the home has an impact, however subtle, on our ability to rest and regenerate. The proposal to create a "house of sleep" is not to turn the home into a silent, rigid monastery, but to infuse domestic life with greater awareness about the importance of deceleration, mutual respect, and creating an atmosphere that nourishes body and soul. This transformation begins with individual awareness but flourishes through dialogue and collaboration among residents. It's an invitation to collectively rethink: how can we make our home a place that truly supports our rest and well-being? What small adjustments in routine, organization, or communication can contribute to quieter nights for everyone? By engaging in this process, we not only improve our own sleep but also contribute to creating a healthier, more harmonious, and welcoming domestic environment, where rest is valued as an essential part of family life and shared well-being.

Expanding the concept of rest beyond the bedroom is, deep down, an exercise in affective responsibility towards the space we inhabit and the people coexisting within it. The "house of sleep" isn't just a quieter, more organized, or aesthetically welcoming house—it's a home where care translates into daily attitudes, small kindnesses building an emotionally safe atmosphere. It's where one understands that rest isn't absence of movement, but presence of attention; that slowing down at night isn't a luxury, but a gesture of mutual respect. In this sense, cultivating an environment favoring sleep is also a way of saying: "I see you," "I care for myself and for us." With this perspective, even the simplest gestures—like lowering one's voice at night, preparing tea for someone who had a hard day, or keeping a soft light on in the hallway—gain transformative power. They communicate that home is a space for listening and welcoming, where everyone's rhythm matters. This doesn't require perfection or drastic changes, but consistency and intention. The house of sleep is born from daily choices making the environment an ally of well-being, not an obstacle. And the more this care takes root in the routine, the less it becomes an obligation and the more it becomes culture—a natural way of being together, in harmony with rest. After all, a house favoring sleep is, above all, a house where one learns to pause. And in this pausing, there is space for encounter, listening, silent affection sustaining the deepest bonds. Creating a house of sleep is building a home where every night is an invitation to surrender, regeneration, and the trust that, by resting, we are also strengthening what is most essential: belonging and the peace of being at home, inside and out.

Chapter 31
Autonomy and Choices

We arrive at a crucial point in our shared journey through the art of sleeping well. We have come a long way, from understanding the fundamental value of sleep to exploring its complex architecture, its intrinsic relationship with health, the barriers modern life imposes, and the beliefs that limit us. We delved into a rich universe of practical techniques, learning to manage our environment, our breath, our body, our senses, our mind, and even our nutrition to cultivate deeper rest. We explored the historical, cultural, and symbolic dimensions of sleep, recognizing its therapeutic strength and creative potential. Now, on the threshold of concluding this path, the invitation is for you to fully take the reins of your own relationship with sleep, integrating all the acquired knowledge and recognizing your innate ability to make conscious choices to nurture your well-being. This chapter is a synthesis and, at the same time, a rite of passage: the moment you cease being a student of this course to become your own guide, the master of your own art of resting.

Throughout these pages, we aimed to offer a comprehensive map of the sleep territory, presenting a variety of tools and perspectives. However, it's crucial to reinforce an essential truth: there are no universal magic formulas or one-size-fits-all solutions. Every human being is unique, with their own biology, life history, sensitivities, challenges, and needs. What works wonderfully for one person may not have the same effect on another. The techniques and strategies presented are like a menu of possibilities, a set of resources you can draw upon, experiment with, and adapt to your individual reality. True mastery lies not in rigidly applying all suggestions, but in developing the wisdom to discern what is most beneficial for you at each moment.

This wisdom is born from the consolidation of three fundamental pillars permeating our entire journey: self-knowledge, listening to the body, and creating coherent habits. Self-knowledge, cultivated through personal diagnosis, the sleep diary, reflection on limiting beliefs, and careful observation of your reactions to different practices, is the foundation upon which you will build your individualized path. Knowing your patterns, sensitivities, stress triggers, and specific rest needs is what allows you to make informed and effective choices.

Listening to the body is the compass that will guide you on this journey. Learning to recognize subtle signs of tiredness, requests for relaxation, feelings of comfort or discomfort regarding the environment, temperature, or food is crucial. Your body possesses innate intelligence and is constantly communicating with you. Honoring this communication, responding to signs of drowsiness by preparing for rest, adjusting room temperature when feeling cold or hot, choosing foods that nourish without weighing you down, means re-establishing a relationship of trust and respect with your own physiology. Attentive listening to the body frees you from the tyranny of external rules and connects you with your inner wisdom.

Creating coherent habits is what transforms knowledge into sustainable practice. Consistency in applying nightly rituals, maintaining regular schedules, practicing relaxation techniques, or managing the luminous environment is what allows the body and mind to adapt and reap long-term benefits. However, coherence does not mean inflexible rigidity. It means creating a support structure that works for you most of the time, but with the necessary flexibility to adapt to life's inevitable variations, as we explored when discussing cycles and seasons. It's about building a lifestyle where sleep care is integrated naturally and fluidly, not as a burden, but as an expression of your commitment to well-being.

With these tools – self-knowledge, body listening, and coherent habits – you are now fully equipped to exercise your autonomy. You have the power to choose which techniques to incorporate into your ritual, which foods to avoid at night, how to adapt your room, when to seek extra rest moments, how to respond to specific challenges that may arise. You understand that sleep isn't something that just "happens" to you, but something you actively cultivate through your daily decisions. Every choice, however small – turning off the light a bit earlier, dedicating five minutes to conscious breathing, opting for a calming tea instead of alcohol – is a brick in building more restorative nights and fuller days.

This perception elevates sleep to a new level of meaning. It ceases to be just a biological function and becomes something sacred, a time of withdrawal and renewal deserving honor and protection. Caring for sleep becomes an act of reverence for life, a recognition of our interconnection with natural rhythms, and a profound expression of self-love. The daily decisions we make regarding our rest become conscious choices reflecting our values and commitment to a more balanced and meaningful life.

This is the moment of your autonomy. You hold the knowledge, the tools, and, most importantly, the ability to observe, adapt, and choose what is best for you. The pages of this book served as a guide, but the journey, from here on, is yours. Trust your intuition, your body's wisdom, and your capacity to learn and grow. Be patient with yourself on difficult days and celebrate every small victory. Remember that the art of sleeping well, like any art, is a continuous process of practice, refinement, and discovery. You are the artist of your own night, the master of your own rest. Embrace this responsibility and power with joy and confidence, knowing that by caring for your sleep, you are caring for your life in its entirety.

Recognizing that autonomy is the pinnacle of this journey, we also realize it doesn't demand perfection, but presence. It's not about always getting it right, but about being willing to reassess and adjust one's path gently. Nights when sleep doesn't come as expected don't nullify the progress made; they just remind us of life's dynamic nature. What matters is the silent, constant commitment to return to oneself, listen to the body again, fine-tune one's rituals, resume the path without guilt, but with awareness. Sleep, after all, is a cycle, and our relationship with it also moves in waves: sometimes calm, sometimes more turbulent, but always alive and transforming.

This art of conducting one's own rest also involves valuing others' autonomy. In a world often imposing standards and ready-made answers, the courage to create a personal style of self-care inspires and liberates. Sleeping well then becomes an act of resistance against the logic of exhaustion and productivity at all costs. By respecting your rhythms, you establish a territory of inner peace where external pressures lose strength, and your authenticity flourishes. In this state of balance, night ceases to be just the end of the day and becomes the beginning of a more integral, present, and free way of living.

And so, sleep ceases to be merely the subject of a study or the target of a quest. It integrates into daily life as a silent ally, a force that sustains, regenerates, and inspires. Knowledge transforms into practical wisdom, and practice into constant care. From here on, each night will be a blank canvas, each choice, a brushstroke. With serenity and autonomy, you will continue, not just as someone who sleeps better, but as someone awakening to a more conscious life—night after night, day after day.

Chapter 32
Sleep Ceremony

Our long and deep journey through the art of sleeping well reaches its final chapter. Together, we unveiled the mysteries of sleep, faced the barriers distancing us from it, explored an arsenal of practical tools, and cultivated a new awareness about the vital importance of rest. You have walked a path of self-knowledge, experimentation, and transformation, assuming autonomy over your nights and, consequently, over your days. To mark the conclusion of this learning cycle and, more importantly, to consecrate the beginning of a new cycle of conscious sleep in your life, we now propose a moment of celebration and commitment: a sleep ceremony. This is not a prescribed ritual, but an invitation for you to create your own symbolic celebration, an intentional act to honor your journey, recognize your achievements, and affirm your purpose to continue cultivating this art daily.

Every significant transformation deserves recognition and celebration. Throughout this course, you invested time, energy, and attention in one of the most fundamental aspects of your health and well-being. You challenged old beliefs, tried new practices, observed your patterns honestly, and likely already started reaping the benefits of more restorative rest. The sleep ceremony is an opportunity to pause and acknowledge this effort and progress. It's a moment to congratulate yourself for the dedication and courage to seek a more harmonious relationship with yourself and your natural rhythms. Celebrating is not just an act of joy, but also a powerful positive reinforcement, anchoring new learnings and strengthening motivation to continue on the chosen path.

How to create your sleep ceremony? The beauty of this practice lies in its complete personalization. It can be simple or elaborate, brief or more extensive, performed individually or shared with someone trusted. What matters is that it's meaningful to you and reflects your unique journey. Choose a quiet time, perhaps at dusk or on a weekend morning, in a place where you feel at peace – it could be your sanctuary-bedroom, a special corner of the house, or even a place in nature. Prepare the environment with elements conveying serenity: a candle, soft incense, calm music, flowers, objects symbolizing your journey.

The heart of the ceremony can include different elements, inspired by the practices explored throughout the book. Gratitude is a powerful starting point. Dedicate time to reflect and perhaps write or verbalize your gratitude for everything learned, the tools discovered, difficulties overcome, and benefits already experienced in your health and well-being. Thank your body for its resilience and healing capacity. Thank sleep itself, recognizing it as a sacred gift.

Defining intentions for the future is another important component. What do you wish to carry forward from this journey? How do you intend to continue cultivating the art of sleeping well in your daily life? Which practices have become most valuable to you, and how can you ensure their continuity? Write down your intentions or state them aloud, clearly and confidently. It could be the intention to continue prioritizing your rest, maintain attentive listening to your body, keep exploring your dreams, or be kinder to yourself in moments of difficulty. These intentions function as seeds planted for the new cycle beginning.

Meditation can be integrated into the ceremony as a moment of stillness, presence, and inner connection. You can do a mindfulness meditation, focusing on breath and the feeling of gratitude, or a guided visualization, imagining yourself enjoying deep, restorative sleep and waking with vitality and clarity. Allow yourself to simply be, absorbing the peace of the moment and the sense of accomplishment.

Writing can also have its place. You might reread significant passages from your sleep diary, recognizing your evolution. You could write a letter to yourself, celebrating your journey and reaffirming your commitments. Or you might simply record the feelings and insights arising during the ceremony.

Consider including a symbolic gesture marking the transition. It could be lighting a candle representing new awareness, planting a seed symbolizing continuous cultivation, drinking calming tea with intention, or any other act holding personal meaning for you. Symbolism helps anchor the experience on a deeper level.

Finally, the ceremony can conclude with an invitation to share. The knowledge and experience you've acquired are valuable not only for yourself but can also inspire and help others struggling with sleep. Reflect on how you can authentically and respectfully share what you've learned with friends, family, or your community. Becoming an agent of change, even on a small scale, spreading awareness about the importance of sleep and practices favoring it, is a way to multiply the benefits of your own journey and contribute to a healthier, more balanced culture. Remember, however, that personal example is the most powerful form of teaching.

This sleep ceremony, your symbolic graduation from this course, does not represent an endpoint, but a milestone. It's the formal recognition that you now possess the tools, knowledge, and autonomy to navigate your relationship with sleep consciously and intentionally. It represents the understanding that sleeping well is not an innate gift or a matter of luck, but an art learned, cultivated, and honored daily, through small choices and consistent practices. And by creating this ceremony, you celebrate not only sleep but also yourself as someone who chose to care with presence and depth for one of life's most fundamental facets.

This intimate and symbolic gesture inaugurates a new stage: living rest as part of your own way of being in the world. With each lit candle, each pronounced intention, each conscious breath, you strengthen the bond with this art now belonging to you, not as theory or technique, but as lived knowledge. The ceremony marks this threshold: from someone seeking answers, to someone who has come to trust listening to the body, the wisdom of silence, the strength of simple yet transformative rituals.

Allow this moment to reverberate. Let it not fade with the end of a chapter, but unfold into your future nights, imbuing them with meaning and presence. By welcoming sleep as a sacred space, you offer yourself the chance to rest not just the body, but also the agitated mind, unsaid fears, pressing urgencies. Sleeping, in this new understanding, is also an act of loving surrender to life as it is. A surrender not demanding perfection, just availability. A practice renewed night after night, like a continuous dialogue between you and the regenerating mystery of repose.

Thus, the journey transforms into a path, and the path becomes part of who you are. May your sleep ceremony be the beginning of a deep and gentle commitment to your inner peace. May you return to it whenever you need reminding why you started, and where you want to go. And may each night, from now on, be lived as a new invitation—silent, tender, and essential—to care for yourself with the same presence with which, until now, you have cared for sleep. Because, deep down, resting well is also a way of loving yourself whole.

Epilogue

Perhaps, when starting this reading, you were looking for answers. Perhaps you wanted to understand why your body rests but doesn't recover, why your thoughts seem louder at night than during the day. Or perhaps you came moved by a silent intuition: that there was something to be reclaimed within yourself.

If that was the case—well, you have reached the end. And, at the same time, the beginning.

This book did not intend merely to teach you how to sleep better. It proposed a reunion. A delicate return to your rhythmic, cyclical, sensitive nature. Throughout the pages, you learned that sleep is more than a physiological function: it is a gesture of trust. A daily surrender only possible when there is safety, presence, and peace.

You understood that sleeping well depends not only on the quiet of the room but on the quiet within. That resting is often *allowing yourself to be*—without performance, without guilt, without urgency. And that each ritual built, however simple it seems, is a vow of care for yourself.

Now, as you close this book, something important needs to be said: your body heard everything. Every page read, every practice tested, every small change in routine left marks. Maybe you are still at the beginning of this process. Maybe you are already feeling the subtle effects of a truly restful night. Or maybe it will take a little longer. It doesn't matter: you planted something. And sleep is generous to those who plant with patience.

There will be no perfection. There will be difficult nights, setbacks, forgetfulness. But there will also be—and above all—a new perspective. A new pact with your own existence. And this pact, however silent, changes everything. It changes how you work, eat, love, be in the world.

May you carry with you, from now on, not just the techniques, but the essence: rest as a right, ritual as a bridge, sleep as healing. May every sunset be an opportunity for return, not exhaustion. And may, each night, you lie down with less hurry, less weight... and more presence.

The world will keep rushing. But now you know there is another possible rhythm. Your rhythm.

Turn off the lights. Breathe deeply. The night is not an enemy—it's shelter.

Sleep well.

www.ingramcontent.com/pod-product-compliance
Lightning Source LLC
Chambersburg PA
CBHW031348230926
51848CB00002B/433